COMMUNICATING WITH
NEUROLOGICAL PATIENTS:
THE NURSE'S ROLE

D0276375

Biomedical Library
Queen's University Belfast
Tel: 028 9097 2710
E-mail: BiomedicalLibrary@qub.ac.uk

For due dates and renewals:

QUB borrowers see 'MY ACCOUNT' at
http://library.qub.ac.uk/qcat
or go to the Library Home Page

HSC borrowers see 'MY ACCOUNT' at
www.honni.qub.ac.uk/qcat

This book must be returned not later
than its due date but may be recalled
earlier if in demand

Fines are imposed on overdue books

COMMUNICATING WITH NEUROLOGICAL PATIENTS: THE NURSE'S ROLE

Talking to People who Have Neurological Disorders or Disabilities

MARGOT LINDSAY RGN BA ALA

Staff Nurse, Outpatients Department,
The National Hospital for Nervous Diseases,
Queen Square, London; Formerly Research Assistant,
National Society for Epilepsy Chalfont Centre,
Chalfont St Peter, Buckinghamshire

Foreword by

THE BARONESS COX OF QUEENSBURY FRCN

Scutari Press
London

© Scutari Press 1990
A division of Scutari Projects Ltd, the publishing company of the
Royal College of Nursing

First published 1990

British Library Cataloguing in Publication Data
Lindsay, Margot
    Communicating with neurological patients: the nurse's role.
    1. Neurological patients. Nursing
    I. Title
    610.7368

    ISBN 1-871364-37-X

Typeset, printed and bound by the Alden Press, Osney Mead, Oxford

CONTENTS

FOREWORD

'Doing the neuro obs'... How many times will nurses find themselves charged with this responsibility from the earliest days of their professional career? But how often do we stop to think of the human reality that lies behind those observations − of the meaning of the condition that requires them? How much do we know about the physical, psychological and social implications of the patient's predicament? How much better could we help those who depend on us if we knew and understood more.

Here is a book that answers these questions. It is a remarkable achievement, interweaving knowledge and insight, scientific fact and telling accounts of the human poignancy of the reality of neurological disorders. It is also a resource book with practical advice ranging from the skills of assessment interviews to basic information on neurophysiology and neuropathology. It differentiates myth from fact. Nurses are given the necessary information to enable them to answer questions accurately, or it may help them to have the confidence to listen sensitively − for such 'masterly inactivity' can be an equally appropriate and challenging therapeutic response.

In achieving these diverse objectives Margot Lindsay has clearly drawn on her extensive nursing experience: her book thus bears all the hallmarks of being written by a nurse for nurses. It is a very competent professional synthesis of knowledge drawn from the clinical and the social sciences, focusing on the challenges facing nurses as they help each individual patient to adjust to the challenge, and often the tragedy, of neurological disorder or disease.

I therefore welcome and wholeheartedly recommend this book. I do so as a nurse who has also studied and taught social science. I am, therefore, perhaps entitled to express this concern about recent developments in nursing education − a concern that I know is shared by some of my nurse colleagues. It is the worry that, in the attempt to broaden the curriculum away from excessive dependence on medical science and in the praiseworthy endeavour to ensure that we see patients as people and not as diseases, we run a risk of undervaluing the clinical sciences. This book splendidly corrects such a trend. As I have already emphasised, it combines both the necessary clinical knowledge of disease and the dimension of the human experience of that disease. The case studies in the final chapter enable the reader to have some 'feeling' of the fears, the sense of stigma, the practical and social problems that are inherent parts of the illnesses underlying the diagnostic labels.

I believe that no nurse who reads Margot Lindsay's book will ever 'do the neuro obs' in quite the same way again. As people who need 'neuro obs' are found in many of the places where nurses work, I hope that every nurse who works in those areas will read it. I can assure you that it is amazingly readable. One can rarely say of a textbook that it is hard to put down, but I did find myself so engrossed that I missed my lunch-break! Need I say more than that? Margot Lindsay has given us a valuable resource book not only in its rich resources for all who work with neurological patients, but in its example of how to combine so many different kinds of knowledge in ways that can truly enhance the quality of nursing practice. I do indeed need to say no more than that – for that is the ultimate objective of all our professional endeavours.

Caroline Cox

PREFACE

Most nurses manage to complete their training with only a vague idea of what neurology is. Doing the 'neuro obs' on head-injured patients reminds us of the importance of neurological status, but apart from encounters with patients who have Parkinson's disease, cerebrovascular disease or epilepsy, neurology is usually regarded as an esoteric subject to be left to doctors. There is an abundance of literature on neurology for the medical profession, but the nurse's own ignorance of the subject is reflected by an enormous gap in the nursing literature. The existing nursing texts focus on the acute problems of the hospitalised patient and seldom consider the lifelong adjustment required by someone who has to live with a neurological disorder.

The aim of the book is to provide a basic introductory text to enable the nurse who is unfamiliar with neurology to talk to her patients in an informed manner. In the past, doctors and nurses were reluctant to mention some neurological conditions and frank discussion of facts was avoided. Furtive consultation by patients of often out-of-date textbooks and medical encyclopaedias led to horrific and inaccurate notions of the illness. However, vivid presentations in the media may be over-dramatised and some equally frightening and popular alternative medicine literature provides dogmatic, biased or incorrect information about cures, which errs on the side of optimism.

The root cause of much fear and anxiety is the lack of understanding among those who have to live with a neurological disorder. The best antidote to fear is increased knowledge and understanding of the condition in its wider aspects. The deeper one's knowledge, the easier it is to get a particular problem into perspective. Patients want to know why they have a particular disease, what they can and should do about it and what will happen to them in the future. Lack of answers to these questions can be the worst part of being labelled a sufferer from a neurological disorder.

Much of the information needed for the care of patients in hospital can be found in this book, but the nurse also has to work from the patient's experience of living with the disorder at home, which can be difficult for the hospital-based practitioner. The decision about how much and what depth of information will be helpful to patients is determined by each individual patient's situation and it is important to avoid giving information that would conflict with what the doctor has said to him.

Some patients will worry about their job, others will be concerned about the effects of disability on their close relatives and friends, while others will be largely worried about their changing body image, but it is the patient himself who will focus our attention on his problem.

Margot Lindsay
1989

In the interests of clarity and to avoid infelicities of phraseology, the convention that nurses are female and patients are male, except where the context dictates otherwise, has been adopted throughout this book.

ACKNOWLEDGEMENTS

My greatest debt is to Sister M Swann and nursing colleagues in the Outpatients Department at Queen Square who have tolerated my endless 'projects' with infinite patience and kindness. I appreciate the constant encouragement provided by Drs Simon Shorvon, Jolyon Oxley and Linda Luxon. Valuable textual criticism has come from Geoff Blackie and Renatta Whurr. I am most grateful for the technical advice about electrophysiological tests from Dr Murray and his team: Alison Polglase, Sarah Ingerfield, Anita Pheby, Mary Boland and Ed Hooke in the EEG Department. To my editor, Patrick West, I owe a large debt for all his painstaking assistance and encouragement. My warmest appreciation is reserved for all those patients who have talked to me about their experiences of living with neurological disorders and, in particular, to Reg Wheeler whose three illustrations make the book much more friendly than otherwise possible.

ML

To Jeremy Holmes and Adelaide Schweitzer, with gratitude

GLOSSARY

This Glossary contains only those terms that are not adequately defined in the text (please refer to the index) or which the trained nurse could be expected to know.

Abduct From the Latin *abducere* meaning 'drawing away', used to name structures that move away from the middle line of the body. The abducens, or VIth cranial nerve, supplies the lateral rectus muscle that 'draws away' the eyeball to the side of the head.

Acuity Clarity or clearness, especially of the vision.

Adduction Movement towards the medial aspect of the body.

Afferent or sensory nerves Carry impulses from the periphery to the brain. *See also* **Efferent nerves**.

Agnosia Loss of the power to recognise the impact of sensory stimuli; the varieties correspond with the senses and are distinguished as auditory, visual, olfactory, gustatory and tactile.

Agraphia Inability to express thoughts in writing.

Aneurysm An abnormal sac-like swelling formed by the dilation of the wall of an artery, often where it branches.

Angioma A congenital abnormality formed from abnormal blood vessels, which shunts arterial blood through to veins too quickly, causing cerebral anoxia and a seizure focus.

Anosmia Absence of the sense of smell.

Anoxia Absence of oxygen supply to tissue despite adequate perfusion of the tissue by blood.

Anticoagulant Any substance that suppresses, delays or nullifies coagulation of the blood.

Aphasia Defect or loss of power of expression by speech, writing or sounds or comprehending language.

Aphonia Loss of voice.

Arteriogram An X-ray of an artery after injection of a radio-opaque medium.

Arteriovenous Affecting an artery and a vein.

Asymptomatic Showing or causing no symptoms.

Atonic Lacking normal tone or strength.

Atropine An anticholinergic agent used chiefly as an antispasmodic to relax smooth muscles, to relieve the tremor and rigidity of Parkinsonism and to increase heart-rate by blocking the vagus nerve.

Audiometry Measurement of hearing, by means of an audiometer.

Aura A subjective sensation or motor phenomenon that precedes and marks the onset of a paroxysmal attack, such as an epileptic attack.

Axon That process of a neuron by which impulses travel away from the cell body.

Basal ganglia   Collections of grey nerve cells deep in the white matter of the brain.

Bell's palsy   A peripheral facial paralysis caused by a lesion of the VIIth cranial nerve, named after Sir Charles Bell, a Scottish anatomist who described the condition in 1830.

Benzodiazepines   Antianxiety drugs used to treat psychoneurotic and anxiety disorders, and to relax muscles.

Bilateral   Having two sides, affecting both sides.

Bitemporal   Concerning both temples or temporal bones.

Blood–brain barrier   There is free and rapid passage of substances between the brain and the CSF, but there is a barrier between the blood and the CSF: the blood–brain barrier. This maintains a constant milieu for brain metabolism and is a protection against noxious substances in the circulation.

Bradykinesia   Abnormal slowness in starting and carrying out voluntary movement.

Bruit   A 'slushing' sound or murmur heard in auscultation (with the stethoscope), indicative of blood passing through narrowed or stenosed vessels.

Cerebellar   Relating to the cerebellum.

Cerebellum   The portion of the brain below the cerebrum and above the medulla oblongata. The hind-brain.

Chiasm   An X-shaped crossing. The **optic chiasm** is the part of the hypothalamus formed by the decussation, or crossing, of the fibres of the optic nerve from the medial half of each retina.

Cholinesterase   An enzyme that rapidly destroys the chemical transmitter acetylcholine.

Circle of Willis   A continuous circle of blood vessels at the base of the brain.

Clonus   Alternate muscular contraction and relaxation in rapid succession. Muscle rigidity and relaxation that occurs spasmodically.

Cognition   That operation of the mind by which we become aware of objects of thought or perception; it includes all aspects of perceiving, thinking and remembering.

Cog-wheel rigidity   Rigid muscles respond to slow stretch by steady resistance, but when a series of little jerks occurs this tremor is described as a 'cog-wheel' effect.

Collateral vessels   Normally there is no flow of blood round the Circle of Willis, but if one of its arteries becomes occluded, blood crosses the circle to make good the deficit. Collateral vessels are therefore additional to the cerebral circulation.

Compression of brain   May be due to pressure from a tumour or blood clot.

Concussion   Transient loss of consciousness following severe head injury. It occurs without there being any gross damage to the brain. It may last for a few seconds or a few hours.

Congenital   Applied to conditions existing at or before birth.

Contracture   Fibrosis causing deformity.

Convolutions   Folds or coils of the cerebrum.

Coordination   The ability to maintain a chosen posture and perform accurate voluntary movements.

Corneal reflex   Touching the cornea with a wisp of cotton wool makes the patient blink with both eyes.

Cortex   The external layers of an organ e.g., of the cerebrum.

Corti, organ of   Spiral organ; the organ resting on the basilar membrane in the cochlear duct, which contains the special sensory receptors for hearing.

Corticosteroids   Hormones produced by the adrenal cortex or their synthetic substitutes.

Craniotomy   A surgical opening of the skull made to relieve pressure, arrest haemorrhage or remove a tumour.

Degeneration   Deterioration, especially change of tissue to a lower or less functionally active form. Degenerative diseases may occur either because cells die or because of some failure of their blood supply to maintain their normal nutrition.

Déjà vu   (French: already seen) An illusion in which a new situation is incorrectly viewed as a repetition of a previous situation.

Demyelination   Destruction, removal or loss of the myelin sheath of a nerve or nerves, which interferes with transmission of the impulses along the nerve fibres in the central nervous system.

Disorientation   Inability to appreciate surroundings, time or personal identity.

Disseminated   Scattered or dispersed.

Dorsiflexion   Backward flexion or bending, as of the hand or foot. *See also* **Flexion**.

Dura mater   A strong fibrous membrane, forming the outer covering of the brain and spinal cord.

Dysphonia   Any impairment of voice; a difficulty in speaking. **Spastic dysphponia**: difficulty in speaking due to excessively vigorous adduction of the vocal cords against each other, so that the voice is hoarse, soft and strained.

Dyspnoea   Difficult or laboured breathing.

Dyspraxia   Partial loss of ability to perform coordinated acts.

Efferent or **motor nerves**   Convey impulses from the brain and cord to the periphery.

Empathy   The power of projecting oneself into the feelings of another person or situation.

Encephalitis   Inflammation of the brain.

Endolymph   The fluid inside the membranous labyrinth of the ear. Excess endolymph is present in Menière's disease.

Extension   A stretching or straightening out.

Extensor   A muscle that extends a part.

Extracranial   Outside the cranium.

Extradural   Outside the dura mater.

Extramedullary   Situated or occurring outside any medulla, especially the medulla oblongata.

Extrapyramidal system   Is composed of special fibres arising from the frontal lobes, the basal ganglia and the brainstem and forms a pathway transmitting motor impulses from the brain to the spinal cord. Habitual and automatic activities of the body, such as those dealing with posture and smooth continuous movements of the hands and arms, are mediated by the extrapyramidal system.

Fasiculations   Isolated fine muscle twitches, which give a flickering appearance.

Febrile convulsion   Convulsion that occurs in childhood and is associated with pyrexia.

Flaccid   Soft, flabby. *See also* **Paralysis**.

Flexion   A bending or doubling up.

Flexor   Muscle that flexes a joint.

Frontal   Relating to the forehead.

Ganglia   Plural of ganglion.

Ganglion   A general term for a group of nerve cell bodies located outside the central nervous system, applied to certain nuclear groups within the brain or spinal cord e.g., basal ganglia.

Glia   More than half the brain is occupied by glial tissue. The cells consist of astrocytes and oligodendroglia, the latter being responsible for the formation of myelin around the nerve fibre. Glial cells, unlike nerve cells, are able to regenerate; after injury to the central nervous system, the glial cells replace the damaged nerve cells.

Gyrus   Fold or convolution, especially of the brain. *See also* **Sulcus**.

Haemangioblastoma   A capillary haemangioma of the brain consisting of proliferated blood vessel cells or angioblasts.

Haemangioma   A benign tumour made up of newly formed blood vessels.

Haematoma   A localised collection of blood, usually clotted, in an organ, space or tissue, due to a break in the wall of a blood vessel.

Hemiparesis   Muscular weakness or partial paralysis affecting one side of the body.

Hemiplegia   Paralysis of one side of the body.

Hemisphere   Half of any spherical or roughly spherical structure or organ: e.g. the hemispheres of the brain.

Herpes zoster   Commonly called shingles, an acute, painful inflammatory skin eruption caused by varicella virus in the posterior root ganglion.

Hydrocephalus   A condition marked by dilation of the cerebral ventricles, most often occurring secondarily to obstruction of the cerebrospinal fluid pathways and accompanied by an accumulation of cerebrospinal fluid within the skull; the fluid is usually under increased pressure but occasionally may be of normal pressure or nearly so.

Hypercalcaemia   An excess of calcium in the blood. Manifestations of hypercalcaemia include fatiguability, muscle weakness, depression, anorexia, nausea and constipation.

Hyperthyroidism   Overactivity of the thyroid gland, characterised by increased basal metabolism, goitre and disturbances in the autonomic nervous system.

Hypoglycaemia   An abnormally diminished content of glucose in the blood, which may lead to tremulousness, cold sweat, hypothermia and headache, accompanied by confusion, hallucinations, bizarre behaviour and, ultimately, convulsions and coma.

Idiopathic   Of unknown causation.

Imaging   The production of clarity, contrast and detail in images, especially in radiological and ultrasound images.

Incoordination   Inability to harmoniously adjust the various muscle movements.

Infarction   The formation of an infarct, which is an area of coagulation necrosis in a tissue due to local ischaemia resulting from obstruction of circulation to the area, most commonly by a thrombus or embolus.

Innervation   The distribution or supply of nerves to a part.

Intervertebral   Situated between two vertebrae.

Intracerebellar   Situated within the cerebellum.

Intracranial   Situated within the cranium.

Intradural   Within or beneath the dura.

Intramedullary   Within the spinal cord or medulla oblongata.

Lability   Quick change of expression of mood or feelings.

Labyrinth   The internal ear consists of several cavities called the bony labyrinth, with a series of channels lined with the membranous labyrinth and containing the fluid endolymph as well as the nerve endings for hearing and balance. *See also* **Endolymph**.

Lesion   (Latin: *laesio*, an attack or injury) A injury, wound or morbid structural change in a tissue or organ.

Lobes   See **Fissures**.

Lower motor neurones   Begin as cell bodies in the anterior horn of the spinal cord, pass out in the anterior root of a spinal nerve to be distributed to the periphery, ending in a motor organ of a muscle.

Malformation   Defective or abnormal formation or deformity, especially one acquired during development.

Medulla   A general term for the innermost portion of an organ or structure.

Medulla oblongata   The truncated cone of nerve tissue continuous above with the pons and below with the spinal cord: it contains ascending and descending tracts and important collections of nerve cells that deal with vital functions such as respiration, circulation and special senses.

Meninges   The three membranes that envelop the brain and spinal cord: the dura mater, pia mater and arachnoid.

Motor functioning   Alterations in muscle strength and tone, posture, muscle coordination, reflexes and abnormal movements, which can indicate impaired ability to move.

Myelin   A lipoprotein membrane that winds around the axon of the nerve fibre in a spiral pattern to form the myelin sheath and serves as an electrical insulator for the neurone, enabling impulses to travel along the fibre much faster than is possible in demyelinated fibres.

Myotonia   Lack of muscle tone. A myotonic disease causes slow relaxation and tonic spasm of muscles.

Neural   Relating to a nerve or nerves.

Neurofibromatosis   A familial condition characterised by developmental changes in the nervous system, muscles, bones and skin and the formation of multiple pedunculated soft tumours (neurofibromas) distributed over the entire body, associated with areas of pigmentation. (Also called: multiple neuroma, neuromatosis, and von Recklinghausen's disease)

Neuroglia   The supporting structure of nervous tissue. It consists of a fine web of tissue enclosing peculiar branched cells known as *glial cells.*

Neuroleptic   (Greek *neuron*, nerve+Greek *lepsis*, a taking hold.) Modifying psychotic behaviour, any drug that favourably modifies psychotic symptoms. (Also called antipsychotic and major tranquilliser.) Side-effects of these drugs include involuntary movements and other neurological symptoms.

Neuroma   A tumour or new growth largely made up of nerve cells and nerve fibres.

Neuromuscular system   The arrangement in which muscles and nerves work together.

Neuroreceptor   One of the terminal elements of a dendrite, which receives the stimulus from the neurotransmitter of the adjoining neurone.

Neurosyphilis   Syphilis of the central nervous system.

Neurotransmitter   A substance that is released from the axon terminal of a presynaptic neurone on excitation. It travels across the synaptic cleft to either excite or inhibit the target cell.

Nystagmus   Involuntary rapid movement of the eyeball, which may be horizontal, vertical, rotatory or mixed, i.e. of two varieties. **Gaze nystagmus**   Nystagmus made apparent by looking to the right or left. **Jerky nystagmus**   A slow movement in one direction. Specific types of nystagmus may indicate a lesion anywhere from the inner ear to the vestibular nuclei and their brain stem connections.

Occlusion   An obstruction or a closing off.

Oculomotor   (*Oculo*+Latin *motor*, mover.) Relating to movements of the eye.

Organ of corti   *See* Corti, organ of.

Otosclerosis   (*Oto*+Greek *sklērōsis*, hardening.) A pathological condition of the body labyrinth of the ear, in which there is formation of spongy bone. This causes bony ankylosis of the stapes, and results in conductive hearing loss. Cochlear otosclerosis may also develop, resulting in sensorineural hearing loss.

Ototoxic   Having a deleterious effect upon the VIIIth (acoustic) nerve, or upon the organs of hearing and balance.

Palsy   *See* **Bell's palsy**; *See also* **Paralysis.**

Papilloedema   Swelling of the optic disc seen with the ophthalmoscope, most commonly due to increased intracranial pressure, malignant hypertension or thrombosis of the central retinal vein. Inflammation of the optic nerve (optic neuritis) also causes papilloedema.

Paralysis   Loss of sensation and the power of movement of any part, as the result of interference with the nerve supply. *See also* **Todd's paralysis**.

Parietal   Relating to or located near the parietal bone, as for the parietal lobe. This extensive area of the brain cannot be related to specific parts of the body. It is responsible for the interpretation and correlation of sensation.

Phonation   The utterance of vocal sounds.

Photosensitive   Exhibiting an abnormally heightened reactivity to light. People who are photosensitive to television experience an epileptic seizure.

Prolactinoma   A pituitary tumour that secretes the hormone prolactin.

Prophylactic   Tending to ward off disease; prophylactic medication can prevent migraine attacks.

Pseudobulbar palsy   A spastic weakness of the facial muscles, the muscles of mastication, the tongue and palate. The tongue lies stiffly in the floor of the mouth and there is a spastic dysarthria. Motiveless crying or laughter frequently accompanies a pseudobulbar palsy.

Pyramidal tracts   Where impulses travel in descending tracts from the cerebral cortex to the spinal cord.

Radiculitis   Inflammation of the spinal nerve roots.

Radio-opaque   Not permitting the passage of radiant energy, such as X-rays, the representative areas appearing light or white on the exposed film.

Raised intracranial pressure   The brain, meninges, blood vessels and cerebrospinal fluid are contained within the rigid bony skull. An increase in the volume of intracranial contents raises the pressure; and is identified by a deteriorating level of consciousness, altered pupillary responses, respiratory changes, bradycardia, blood pressure changes, elevated body temperature, headache, vomiting and papilloedema. Common causes are an expanding neoplasm, abscess or cerebral haemorrhage, and oedema caused by inflammatory disease or trauma.

Receptor   A receptor nerve ending is the sensory terminal that receives and registers stimuli from its environment.

Retro   In anatomy 'retro' refers to behind in space, as in **retrobulbar** meaning the space behind the eyeball, which resembles in shape, a medium-sized 'onion' (Latin *bulbus*).

Retrovirus   A large group of RNA (messenger) viruses.

Schwann cell   Any of the large nucleated cells whose cell membrane spirally enwraps the axons of myelinated peripheral neurones and is the source of myelin. Theodor Schwann, German anatomist and physiologist (1810–1882).

Sensory   The brain receives messages from the sensory nerve endings in the skin and these bring information relating to sensations of touch, temperature and pain. A **sensorineural** sign or symptom is related to a sensory nerve.

Shunt   To turn to one side, to divert, to bypass. A surgically created anastomosis. Arteriovenous shunt – a direct passage of blood from an artery to a vein.

Spondylitis   Is an inflammation of a vertebra, from the Greek word *spondylos*, a vertebra.

Sternocleidomastoid   Relating to the sternum, clavicle and mastoid process.

Sternomastoid   Pertaining to the sternum and the mastoid process of the temporal bone.

Steroid   In addition to the naturally occurring hormones hydrocortisone and cortisone, a number of synthetic steroids are used therapeutically, e.g. prednisone, prednisolone and aldosterone. All patients having steroids must carry drug cards containing details of their treatment and warning notices.

Subarachnoid   Situated or occurring between the arachnoid and the pia mater.

Substantia nigra   Beneath the thalamus a narrow band of nerve cells whose colour is much darker than the usual grey because of a pigment derived from the neurotransmitter dopamine contained within the cells.

Sulcus   An almost endless variety of grooves, depressions and wrinkles in anatomic structures have been called a sulcus, or in the Latin plural, *sulci*.

Synapse   (Greek *synaptō*, 'I join together'.) The term describes connection between the processes of two nerve cells.

Syncope   A transient loss of consciousness due to cerebral ischaemia. The onset is gradual and preceded by feelings of weakness, dizziness, nausea, hazy vision and sweating. The patient slips limply to the ground and seldom injures himself. He is pale and his pulse is of strong volume. If allowed to lie flat, recovery occurs after a minute or two and is usually gradual, like the onset.

Syndrome   A group of symptoms or signs that run together as characteristic of a given condition.

Systemic   Relating to a whole system or several systems.

Todd's paralysis   Transient paralysis following an epileptic seizure. It usually lasts only a few minutes or hours, and if lasting more than 48 hours, requires careful medical investigation.

Two-point discrimination   This tests the patient's sensation of touch. The normal individual can distinguish the two points of a pair of dividers from 2 to 4 mm apart when they are pressed on to the pulp of his finger. The accuracy varies from individual to individual and over different parts of the body.

INTRODUCTION

The text of Chapter 1, *Observing the Patient and Assessing his Problems*, is organised according to the nurse's interaction with patients, in which she observes, assesses and listens to what they have to say about their difficulties. Participation in the neurological examination will help the nurse to recognise the physiological changes in neurological disorders. The more emotionally demanding themes of diagnosis – listening to the patient, and the carer's feelings – are introduced in this chapter. Having observed how a person moves, sits or stands and communicates with people around him, the nurse can then identify the most common problems experienced by the patient, as described in Chapter 2, *Problems Experienced by Patients*. The nurse who meets a patient with dementia, a speech disorder, hearing loss, mobility problems, pain, dysphagia or sexual difficulties caused by a neurological disorder will find some useful information in the second chapter.

Chapter 3, *Nurse's Core Information*, provides the nurse with basic facts about neurological conditions: cerebrovascular disorders, degenerative, movement and epileptic disorders as well as dementing diseases, tumours and the myasthenic syndromes.

The long-term needs of the patient coping with a neurological disorder and the attitudes of nurses are considered in Chapter 4, *Psychosocial Aspects of Neurological Disorders*. There are few cures in neurology. The doctor provides medical care for the patient to alleviate his symptoms of rigidity, muscle spasm, involuntary movements or sphincter problems, for example, and the nurse can offer psychosocial support through an informed relationship; however, she will need to be aware of her attitudes towards selected patient groups as well as to the stigma of disability.

Some factual data provided in Chapter 5, *Living with a Neurological Disorder*, help to answer patients' questions about who contracts a neurological disorder, reasons for investigative procedures and the patient's fears. Case studies described in this chapter are based on accumulated experiences compiled from a number of neurological patients.

Using the book

After meeting the patient and assessing his problems (Chapters 1 and 2), the nurse can then refer to other chapters in the book as the need arises: sometimes she will need an overall picture of a disorder (Chapter 3); on other occasions she will want to know the incidence of specific syndromes (Chapter 5); and there will be times when thinking about and discussing the psychosocial aspects of neurological disease will be most relevant (Chapter 4). At any time she may need to see some examples of patients' experiences (Chapter 5). It is to be hoped that the book will prove sufficiently stimulating for the reader to be encouraged to look into neurological nursing in depth with the help of references and further reading. Sometimes patients' questions are impossible to answer, which is something with which the nurse involved with neurological patients must come to terms. However, sufficient information will be found in these pages to enable the nurse to talk to neurological patients in an informed way and to gain an understanding of what life is like for them.

Chapter 1

OBSERVING THE PATIENT AND ASSESSING HIS PROBLEMS

Chapter theme

For nurses preparing for patient education and discussions with patients and their relatives, the section entitled 'Feelings and knowledge' in this chapter provides an objective aid to the measurement of attitudes and will help to define areas needing particular attention. A professional relationship is based on acquired knowledge; therefore it is inadequate merely to identify that a patient has mobility or speech problems because of a neurological disorder. The section on 'Activities of daily living' provides objective tools to help to define the patient's disability.

Understanding a patient's symptoms requires at least a basic knowledge of neuroanatomy and physiology; the most practical way of learning this is through participating in the clinical examination. If the nurse queries why the doctor pays particular attention to one area, such as the cranial nerves or the motor system, and then relates this to the patient's symptoms, a lesson in practical neuroanatomy and physiology can be learnt.

It is a critical time for the patient and his family when he learns of his diagnosis, as this may represent a new self-image and identity as a disabled person. The nurse may have to help him sort out the myths of his condition from the facts. When the nurse meets a patient who has an undiagnosed condition she can prepare herself for the discussion by reading the 'Diagnosis' section in this chapter. Patients may be so distracted by anxiety that they are unable to listen to what they hear. Nurses have to have the humility to listen and not to insist on asserting control too soon, if at all; for this they require the development of confidence and strength. The subsection on 'Listening' offers some suggestions for developing this important skill.

To help the general trained nurse to recognise the psychological losses implied by neurological disability, the 'Losses' section points to some questions that the patient may ask that indicate his concerns about a threat to his life-style. Her attention is also drawn to the denial process, an important adjustment phase for the person confronted by a chronic disabling illness.

Contents

Feelings and knowledge

Questions

Headaches

A detailed history of the patient's headaches will enable the doctor to understand the nature and causative factors and help in planning treatment. The information that patients are asked to provide includes the following items:

1. Date of the first episode of a similar headache.
2. Average frequency of attacks per week, month or year.
3. Warning of the onset of the headache.
4. The description of the pain in the patient's own words e.g. dull, throbbing or unbearable.
5. Any known precipitating or aggravating factors.
6. The exact location of the pain – whether it occurs all over the head or is consistently confined to one area.
7. Intolerance of noise, light or odours during an attack.
8. Nausea, vomiting or diarrhoea during or after an attack.
9. Disorders of movement, speech or other sensations before or during an attack.
10. Dizziness, faintness or transient loss of consciousness.
11. How the attacks interrupt normal daily activities.
12. Whether any treatment has already been tried, and its effectiveness.
13. Any known relationship between attacks and the menstrual cycle.
14. Whether or not the person has had similar attacks earlier in life.
15. Whether or not the person has had bilious attacks or travel sickness as a child.
16. Whether or not the patient is taking the contraceptive pill, or whether or not it has influenced the frequency or severity of her headache.
17. Any family history of migraine, which is important background information.

Dizziness

Because of the many different meanings of *dizziness*, specific information about the patient's experiences will be required in order to reach a precise diagnosis of his problems. Appropriate questions could include:

1. Is the dizziness constant or does it occur intermittently?
2. If intermittent, is the patient well between attacks?
3. When did the dizziness first begin?
4. Is there anything that can bring on attacks or aggravate the dizziness (e.g. specific head movements, standing up too quickly)?
5. Is there anything that relieves the dizziness (e.g. lying down, tablets, keeping the head still)?

6. Has the patient ever fallen or had any loss of consciousness?
7. If the patient has attacks of dizziness, how often do these occur and are there any long, clear periods?
8. Are the attacks associated with nausea or vomiting?
9. Are the attacks associated with a feeling of faintness, crumbling sensation of the legs, a feeling of movement or spinning?
10. If there is a spinning sensation, for how long can this last continuously at its worst?
11. Is there any deafness in either ear? Does this fluctuate or associate with the dizziness?
12. Is there any noise (*tinnitus*) in either ear? Does this fluctuate or associate with the dizziness?
13. Is there any feeling of pressure or fullness in either ear? Is this associated with the dizziness?
14. Was the onset of the dizziness associated with any specific event e.g. illness, bereavement?
15. Was the onset of the dizziness associated with any sudden change of pressure in the ear, such as in an aircraft or on suddenly lifting something heavy, or with other forms of exertion or straining?

The patient will also be asked whether or not he has had any headaches, changes in vision or numbness of the face or fingers. There may also be questions about increased clumsiness, problems with breathing during the dizziness or recent weight changes. The presence of ear, blood pressure or heart problems will be relevant, and it is vital for the patient to be able to state what, if any, medication he is currently taking, as this could be a cause of his dizziness. Also important is whether or not the patient has ever been exposed to excessive noise at work or explosive noise as when using a gun: these could be environmental causes of dizziness.

Assessing attitudes

How does the patient view the meaning and significance of his ill-health? How do the patient's family and friends view his ill-health? What explanatory models do they use?

1. What has happened? (labelling the condition)
2. Why has it happened? (aetiology)
3. Why me? (relation to diet, behaviour, personality, heredity)
4. Why now? (timing, mode of onset)
5. What would happen if nothing were done about it? (its likely course, outcome, prognosis and dangers)
6. What should I do about it? (self-treatment consultations with lay advisers or health professionals)

(Helman, 1984).

Attitudes

Pain

Pain is not just a physical sensation, it is also an emotion, which helps to explain the wide variation in its perception. It varies with different people and according to accompanying sensations. The perception of pain is increased by fear, discomfort and pain itself, which explains the importance of preventing pain from occurring, rather than trying to cope with it once it has occurred (Hough, 1986).

If no cause for pain has been found after several attempts at diagnosis, the patient will begin to think that the doctor believes he is not in pain. The doctor's position of having to tell the patient that he can find nothing wrong creates a difficult communication problem for everyone concerned. If nurses also believe that the lack of organic causes means there is nothing wrong, the patient will tell his family and friends, 'They just think I'm making it up, they don't understand.' The fact that pain is a subjective, personal experience that cannot be seen, touched or measured presents insurmountable problems for both basic scientists and clinicians. The nurse's personal value system, experiences of pain and cultural attitudes to acceptable behaviour will determine her evaluation of patients who have long-standing pain syndromes.

Blau (1984) has identified fears aroused in patients by their experiences of migraine. In a survey of 51 women and 24 men attending neurological clinics, 50 patients expressed fears. Fear of death was implied by some patients who talked about their 'head exploding' or fear of a tumour. Three people talked about having 'something wrong with the brain' and two had contemplated suicide when in severe pain. Blau suspected that fear of the symptoms of mental illness was more common than a patient would admit because many patients were too frightened to discuss their innermost fears.

Very often, patients do not like to discuss their pain with others. They feel that nobody wants to hear about aches and pains; other people have their own problems to cope with, no-one likes a complainer and no-one wants to be thought a hypochondriac. To understand how a patient sees his pain the following questions can be asked (Melzack, 1975):

1. What do you feel is the cause of the pain?
2. How has your pain been explained to you?
3. How often in a day do you think about your pain?
4. Are there any situations in which you find that you often think about pain?
5. Are there people with whom you discuss your pain problems? If yes, with whom do you share these problems? How often do they respond and in what way?
6. Has this pain problem affected your feelings about yourself as a person? If yes, how?
7. Does religious faith help you to cope with the pain? If yes, in what way?
8. Are there thoughts, memories or fantasies that you can think about that help you cope with your pain? If yes, can you describe them?
9. What other methods do you use that help you cope with the pain problems?

Epilepsy

1. Is epilepsy a form of emotional disorder?
2. Is it contagious?
3. Do people with epilepsy usually have brain tumours?
4. Is epilepsy often caused by drug abuse?
5. Do people frequently die of epileptic seizures?
6. Do epileptic seizures generally become more severe or more frequent as years go by?
7. Are most people with epilepsy addicted to the medication they take?
8. Can medication be discontinued if the patient has not had a seizure for several months?
9. After a seizure, should extra doses of medication be taken for that day?
10. If a person turns blue when having a seizure, does that mean he is going to die?
11. Is it likely that a person may swallow his tongue during a seizure and suffocate as a result?
12. Should something soft always be put in the person's mouth during a seizure to prevent him from biting his tongue?
13. Is epilepsy a type of emotional breakdown?
14. Are people with epilepsy a greater safety risk than others for employers?
15. Should a person with epilepsy have children?
16. Will the child of a woman who has epilepsy also have seizures?

Disability

What is the meaning of the diagnosis in relation to the patient's personal life? What is his attitude to the treatment? Does he have a disabled or able identity? How will the condition affect his family, mental outlook and work? Looking ahead: problems associated with medication, coping at home, getting through bad patches. Questions (adapted from Maybury and Brewin, 1984) to the patient could include:

1. How did your illness start?
2. How did you feel when you were told the diagnosis?
3. What does it feel like to have your particular health problem?
4. Would you say that you have a physical disability?
5. What happens?
6. How do you manage the disease?
7. What is the worst part of the disease?
8. What is the most embarrassing thing you have experienced with your disability?
9. What effect does your disability have on other people?
10. Are the symptoms of the disorder the same all the time?
11. Does anything make the symptoms worse?
12. Does anything make the symptoms better?

Assessing carers' attitudes (Greene, 1982)

1. Do you ever feel that you can no longer cope with the situation?
2. Do you ever feel that you need a break?
3. Do you ever get depressed by the situation?
4. Has your own health suffered at all?
5. Do you worry about accidents happening to . . . ?
6. Do you ever feel that there will be no end to the problem?
7. Do you find it difficult to get away on holiday?
8. How much has your social life been affected?
9. How much has the household routine been upset?
10. Is your sleep interrupted by . . . ?
11. Has your standard of living been reduced?
12. Do you ever feel embarrassed by . . . ?
13. Do you feel that you cannot entertain visitors?
14. Do you ever get cross and angry with . . . ?
15. Do you ever feel frustrated at times with . . . ?

Activities of daily living

Posture and gait

A neurological disorder may first be suspected by a nurse who observes a change in the patient's *gait* (manner of walking). Normal walking depends on an intact motor, *proprioceptive*, and vestibular system, as well as on normal functioning of the higher centres such as the cerebellum and extrapyramidal system. The patient who has a problem with his sense of balance will move in a specific way that the nurse can readily identify: he will be reluctant to move his head and eyes, particularly if the problem is in the vestibular system (he will tend to look ahead as though he has a stiff neck); he prefers slow head or body movement to eye movement; he walks slowly and stiffly upright with his hands feeling for surrounding support; the wider apart his feet are, the more troublesome the balance problem and he will sit down and stand again very carefully.

Observations should be directed towards the patient's movements, with special attention paid to right–left symmetry, swing of the arms, the distance the feet spread from the mid-line in walking (gait base), reciprocal arm motion in relation to leg movement, stability of the pelvis and shoulders during walking, thoracic stability in side-to-side movement, and placement of the heel followed by controlled placement of the toes on the floor. Accurate identification of the patient's difficulties with walking will help the nurse to identify problems such as the risk of loss of balance, falling and other consequences of immobility, which can seriously damage the quality of the patient's daily life.

Mobility

Do you have difficulty walking?

Starting to walk?   Negotiating doorways or walking in
Climbing stairs and steps?   confined spaces?
                                     Answering the door?

Do you have difficulty in:

Getting in and out of bed?   Turning over in bed?
Reaching and picking things up?   Sitting down and getting up again?
Turning and manoeuvring in bed?   Standing up from sitting?
Managing alone in the lavatory?   Balancing?

How would you describe your style of walking?

I walk normally.   I can only take a few steps without
I walk normal distances but a little slowly.   help.
I walk only limited distances.   I can walk only with help.
                                            I am unable to walk.

Speech

Loss or impairment of speech for any reason is one of the most distressing and frustrating conditions that afflict human beings. This is because daily life is deeply concerned with communication. Loss of speech results in isolation, loneliness, frustration, despair, anger and paranoia, in varying degrees according to the circumstances and the individual afflicted.

If the patient can understand, to what extent can he express his thoughts? Can he speak at all? Does he ever speak explosively? Can the patient suddenly use emotional expletives when he is under stress, or can he sing certain songs or recite the Lord's Prayer? Can he read? Can he count and do arithmetical problems? Does the patient understand news reports on radio or television?

The nurse can discuss the patient's difficulty with specific tasks by referring to the following activities:

Making a telephone call.   Talking to strangers, asking for goods in shops.
Talking to friends.   Buying a ticket for bus or train.
Talking at home.   Talking in other people's homes.
Attending social events.   Speaking in a group of people.

A score of 0–6 could be given for a person's level of speech difficulty:

0   Clear, loud, resonant, easily understood.
1   Beginning of hoarseness with loss of inflection and resonance.

2 Moderate hoarseness and weakness, beginning of dysarthria, hesitancy, stuttering, difficult to understand.
3 Marked harshness and weakness, very difficult to hear and understand.

Disorders of the central nervous system often produce symptoms that interfere with daily life. Assessing a person's disability can be greatly helped by asking specific questions that researchers have formulated for particular disorders (Oxtoby, 1982; Newrick and Langton-Hewer, 1984). Selected questions for patients suffering from either *Parkinson's disease* or *motor neurone disease* can be used by the nurse who needs an objective definition of her patient's problems.

ADL in Parkinson's disease (adapted from Oxtoby, 1982)

Do you have difficulty with:

Doing up buttons and zips?	Writing?
Doing your hair/shaving?	Using switches and handles?
Opening bottles, etc?	Bathing?

Have you experienced problems with any of the following:

Dribbling?	Swallowing?
Dry mouth?	Constipation?
Tiring easily?	Bad memory for recent events?

Does a tremor affect your ability to do certain things?

I can hold a cup normally.
I have a bit of difficulty holding a cup without spilling anything.
I have a lot of difficulty holding a cup without spilling anything.

Assessing activities of daily living in motor neurone disease

Newrick and Langton-Hewer (1984) have devised the following assessment scale for motor neurone disease:

Bulbar function

Swallowing:		Speech:	
Normal	3	Normal	2
Chokes occasionally	2	Slurs	1
Chokes regularly	1	Unintelligible	0
Nasogastric tube	0	*Maximum score*=2	
Maximum score=	3		

Drooling:
  Normal   2
  Occasional   1
  Continuous   0
    Maximum score= 2

Top score for bulbar function=7

Limb function

Bathing:
  Independent   1
  Dependent   0
    Maximum score=1

Dressing:
  Independent   2
  Needs some help 1
  Dependent   0
    Maximum score=2

Feeding:
  Independent or manages most 1
  Dependent   0
    Maximum score=   1

Toilet:
  Independent   2
  Some help needed 1
  Dependent   0
    Maximum score= 2

Mobility:
  Independent for 50 m with or without an aid 3
  As above but needs help of one person   2
  Independent with wheelchair   1
  Immobile   0
    Maximum score=   3

Stairs:
  Independent   2
  Manages with help 1
  Unable to manage 0
    Maximum score= 2

Grooming:
  Independent   1
  Dependent   0
    Maximum score=1

Bed–chair transfer:
  Independent   3
  Manages with minimal help 2
  Needs major help   1
  Has to be lifted   0
    Maximum score=   3

Top score for limb function=15

Care source:
  Independent   3
  Help from family   2
  Outside help   1
  Regular holiday relief 0

Top score for care source= 3

The clinical examination

Medical consultation

The purpose of the medical interview is to gather all the information available from the patient to determine the origin and outbreak of his illness and its course and consequences so far. The consultation also promotes a medically useful patient–doctor relationship. In the usual sequence of a medical consultation, history-taking leads to the physical examination. It is only at this stage that the value of the history becomes apparent because a full neurological examination of a patient can take up to an hour. The nature of the examination is based largely on the patient's description of his problems and any previous illnesses, which enables the doctor to select specific areas of body function to investigate. Most patients benefit from contact with a nurse who can explain the individual nature of the clinical examination.

Important neurological symptoms

Because of concern about his present difficulty, the patient may forget to mention symptoms that could be important to the understanding of his neurological problem, or he might feel that they are too trivial to mention. The doctor will want to know about the occurrence of headache, visual symptoms, deafness, vertigo, abnormalities of sense, smell and taste, weakness and altered sensation in his arms and legs, bladder dysfunction and any alterations of consciousness. He will also be concerned to identify signs of neurological dysfunction such as disordered mentation, personality change, memory loss or confusion. There may also be enquiries about altered libido, sexual dysfunction or menstrual irregularities. The patient and his family may be asked about any difficulty in performing daily motor activities and difficulty with speech, swallowing or chewing, as well as insomnia, drowsiness and sleep disorders. Any evidence of tremors or other involuntary movements may also be investigated.

The patient's facial expression may indicate emotions, depression or hostility, or be one of the characteristic facies of myasthenia gravis or Parkinson's disease. Body symmetry and the patient's ease of walking and sitting can give important early clues to neurological deficits, as does the strength and quality of the handshake. The posture of the patient should be noted, as well as the manner in which the hands are held or used.

In order to appreciate the true significance of a symptom, questions may be asked about its nature: onset, severity, exact form or character, relationship to other events, time, meals or postural change, location in body at onset, change in pattern over time, associated symptoms and what relieves or aggravates the symptoms.

Patients' fears

To the patient the physical examination may be the part of the encounter with the doctor about which he is most apprehensive, since he may fear that it will disclose some unexpected or particularly feared, severe, dangerous, disabling or fatal disease. Patients who have never been physically examined by a doctor may associate pain and discomfort with the physical examination. The mere thought of having to expose their naked body to a strange person is felt by some patients to be most unpleasant. The patient may feel humiliated by having to display some real or imagined bodily defect or deformity because he fears that the doctor will find him repugnant or disgusting.

Setting of the medical consultation

Ideally, the medical consultation and neurological examination will take place in a quiet, warm room. As neurologists traditionally practise in hospitals, the patient will initially be seen in an out-patient department of his local hospital.

The effect of ward rounds on patients can be either positive or negative, depending mainly on the way they are conducted. The ward round should be done informally, in a non-intimidatory manner. Appropriate multi-disciplinary staff interested in a person's problems will be brought together to share their ideas. This provides an impetus to go through notes and think about the patient and his problem, brings everyone up to date, so that important tests are not forgotten or results ignored, provides an opportunity for the medical team to work out the general approach to a patient's problems (this stimulus could mean that someone might come up with a new idea) and provides the opportunity for patients to meet the senior doctor on a regular basis and greatly increase their feeling of security.

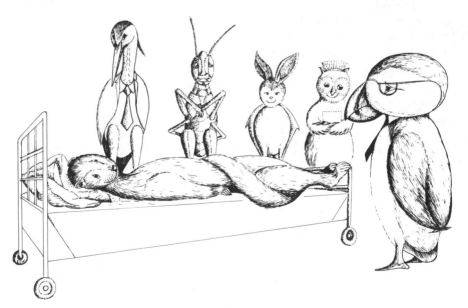

Figure 1.1   The ward round

Review of information about the patient could be discussed prior to the round proper. During the round there should be no more talk about the patient, only with the patient. Information about the patient should always first be sought from himself rather than from staff. The patient should be given the feeling that he is expected to explain how he feels, talk about his symptoms and be free to ask questions. All examination on the rounds should be performed out of sight of other patients. Any discussion following examination should include the patient and the findings should be explained to him in language he can understand. The doctor in charge should if needed, be ready to discuss with the patient, after the round, any matter that may remain unclear. (See also Chapter 1, 'The patient's vocabulary'.) The ward round is one of many memorable experiences for patients in hospital, which may be a focus for creative talent: one patient, Reg Wheeler, expressed his feelings through a series of drawings such as Figure 1.1.

Alternatively, with ward teaching where patients are mobile it is more respectful of the patient's privacy to take him into a side room or consulting room to discuss his case there rather than in the ward where everyone can listen. Case conferences held in a room near the ward in a relaxed, thoughtful atmosphere can teach respect for the patient, and interviewing techniques, and identify gaps between medical and patient use of terms.

Intellectual function

After the medical history has been obtained, the next stage is the neurological examination itself. For every patient this proceeds from the highest level of function to the lowest and from general functions to those which are very specific. A critical factor in assessing a person with dementia-like symptoms is to determine whether or not the symptoms have been caused by a treatable problem. Assessment of dementia can be difficult because of the many factors that one must consider in evaluating a patient with memory loss.

Orientation

The patient is asked if he knows the time of day, week, month and year, if he can name his present location, his name and the names of those around him.

Attention and concentration

A series of numbers is read out and the patient is asked to repeat them: the number of digits in a sequence is increased with each successful repetition by the patient. The patient is then asked to count backwards from 100 by sevens or threes. Healthy people can learn seven numbers forwards and five backwards.

Memory

Retention and immediate recall is assessed by seeing whether the patient can remember the interviewer's name after a 10-minute gap with one or two reminders in the first minutes: this is a useful indication of whether there is a short-term memory difficulty.

Recent memory is tested by asking about events of the previous few days, and immediate recall is gauged by reading a short sentence and asking him to repeat it. Somewhat greater retention is indicated if the patient can successfully recall after 5 minutes a list of a few common objects and a fictitious address or a sentence such as 'There is one thing that a nation must have to be rich and great, and that is a large, secure supply of wood' or 'Tom and Bill went fishing in a river and caught three trout, two salmon and a boot'. Most patients can learn these accurately in three to five attempts; however, the tests are subject to all the problems of anxiety, speech difficulty and memory disturbance. It should be noted here that the results of these tests are not specific for any condition.

Remote memory is assessed through the person's ability to give an account of his life and of his recorded illnesses.

Abstract reasoning

This is assessed by asking the patient to explain the meaning of proverbs: glass houses; rolling stones; strike while the iron is hot. General knowledge tests – the names of public figures, capitals of countries and so on – will all be influenced by the general interests of the patient. Formal psychometric testing is performed by clinical psychologists after referral from neurologists.

The cranial nerves

One of the most compelling aspects of neurological nursing is the detective work required to understand patients' symptoms. Research-oriented nurses can learn much about hypothesis testing by listening to patients explain the various ways by which their problem was investigated until ultimately a diagnosis was reached, sometimes long after the initial presenting symptom. Nevertheless, the most vivid way of experiencing the challenge of neurological assessment is by participating in the examination of the cranial nerves.

Twelve pairs of cranial nerves principally supply the structures of the head and neck (Table 1.1 and Figure 1.2). They are numbered with Roman numerals in the order in which they arise in the brain. Some of them are mainly sensory, e.g. the nerves of the special senses, some are mainly motor and some are mixed, with both motor and sensory fibres. Disease does not pick on one group of fibres alone: many permutations and combinations of abnormalities are possible. Discovering what particular combination is present in the individual patient enables the doctor to determine the site of the lesion and later to identify the specific nature of the disturbance to neurological

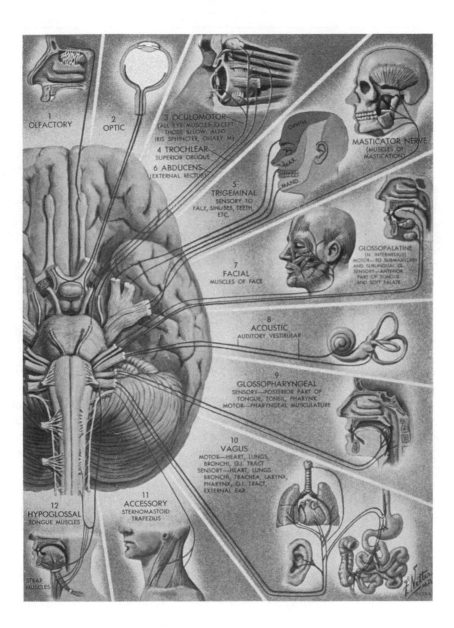

Figure 1.2 The cranial nerves (from *Ciba Collection of Medical Illustrations*, Vol. 1, p. 42. Reproduced by kind permission of Ciba-Geigy plc, Basle, all rights reserved)

Table 1.1 *Cranial nerves*

Number	Name	Function
I	Olfactory	Controls smell
II	Optic	Controls vision
III	Oculomotor	Controls accommodation of the lens, pupillary constriction and the upper eyelid; also controls extraocular movement along with cranial nerves IV and VI
IV	Trochlear	Controls one muscle of the eye: the external oblique
V	Trigeminal	Controls sensation of the face and the muscles of chewing
VI	Abducens	Controls one muscle of the eye: the lateral rectus
VII	Facial	Controls muscles of expression of the face and scalp and taste of the anterior two-thirds of the tongue
VIII	Acoustic	Controls hearing and balance
IX	Glossopharyngeal	Controls taste of the posterior one-third of the tongue; it is tested together with the Xth (vagus) nerve
X	Vagus	Controls larynx, pharynx, vocal cords, swallowing, gag reflexes and taste of the posterior one-third of the tongue
XI	Spinal accessory	Controls movement of the head and neck
XII	Hypoglossal	Controls movement of the tongue

functioning. As each cranial nerve is assessed, both the right and left sides of the head have to be tested.

Disease or injury to the cranial nerves results in the patient experiencing a neurological deficit, e.g. herpes involving the ophthalmic branch of the Vth cranial nerve will be serious if it invades the cornea and results in scarring, which could cause partial or complete blindness. Bell's palsy of the VIIth cranial nerve leaves one side of the patient's face motionless: the eye stays open, tears flow over the face and food accumulates in the cheek, but in most cases the condition resolves. Attacks of stabbing pain lasting from a few seconds to several minutes that occur spontaneously or are produced by talking, eating or washing the face are experienced by the patient with neuralgia of the Vth cranial nerve. Disturbances of the vestibular portion of the VIIIth nerve can lead to vertigo, nausea and vomiting. Signs of abnormality in any of these nerves, even in the absence of symptoms, are important clues in understanding what caused the problems that have brought the patient to the medical consultation.

Neurological examination tray

The following equipment is usually required on an examination tray:

- Ophthalmoscope.
- Auriscope.
- Tongue depressors.
- Patella hammer.
- Reading chart.

- Orange sticks – for superficial reflexes and touch sensation.
- Cotton wool – to test sensation to touch.
- Temperature tubes – hot and cold water tubes for temperature sensation.
- Tuning forks 512 Hz and 128 Hz – to test hearing and vibration sense.
- Pins – to test sensitivity to pain sensation.
- Small torch – to test pupillary response and the gag reflex.
- Tape measure – to measure the cranium or a limb with muscle wasting.
- Stethoscope – to listen for bruits or cardiac disorders and to be used in taking the blood pressure.
- Two-point discriminators – to test differentiation of touch.
- Box of various objects – to test dysphasia: comb, coin, safety pin, key.
- Smelling (cloves and mint) and taste (sugar and salt) samples.
- Red- and white-headed pins – to test visual acuity.
- Ishihara colour vision test book – to test colour vision.

Testing cranial nerve function

I   Olfactory

The olfactory nerve controls the sense of smell. To assess this the patient blocks one nostril and is then asked to sniff strongly and alternately through each nostril, since there are two separate olfactory nerves. He is asked to identify specific smells: peppermint, cloves and lemon. Strong pungent odours such as alcohol, acetone or ammonia should be avoided as these may irritate the patient's nasal mucosa. It is the patient's ability or inability to detect each substance that is important, not whether he can identify it by name.

II   Optic

The optic nerve controls *visual acuity* and the visual fields and it is tested by examination of these functions. When we look at an object, we not only see the object but also a number of other things in the neighbourhood: the full extent of this vision is called the *visual field*. The field of vision is limited by the area of the retina and by the margins of the orbit, nose and cheek. Hence the position of the eye is important.

Loss of sight in half of the visual field is called *hemianopia*. When this is present in the same half of both fields this is described as *homonymous hemianopia*. When the field defect on one side is a mirror image of that on the other, this is said to be *bitemporal* or *binasal*, according to the halves affected. A field defect limited to one quadrant is described as *quadrantic hemianopia*.

Visual acuity is tested by means of standard charts or by the ability to read various sizes of print. Gross visual acuity may be assessed by having the patient count fingers that are held up in front of him.

The retina is inspected through an ophthalmoscope. Of special neurological interest are drooping lids (*ptosis*), protrusion of either eyeball (*proptosis*) and inequalities in the size and shape of the pupils. (See Chapter 5, 'Ronald' and 'Rebecca'.)

III Oculomotor   IV Trochlear   VI Abducens

These three nerves work together to control eye movement and are usually assessed simultaneously.

Pupillary reaction is assessed by asking the patient to fix his eyes on an object and shining a penlight beam directly into each pupil, noting the size, shape and reaction of the pupils to the light stimulus. Under normal circumstances the pupil reacts quickly to light, the contraction being maintained for a brief time and the muscle relaxing as the sphincter of the iris fatigues with continued application of the light.

To assess ocular movement the patient is asked to keep his head still and follow with his eyes the movements of the examiner's finger or a pin upwards, downwards and to either side and to report any experience of double vision (*diplopia*). The position of the eyeballs at rest, any defect of movement and their position when diplopia occurs, can indicate which of these nerves may be injured. (See Chapter 5, 'Rosemary'.)

V Trigeminal

The trigeminal cranial nerve has both sensory and motor functions. It controls jaw movement and the reaction of the face and scalp to pain, temperature and light touch. Symmetrical muscle movement is tested by the examiner placing his hands at the patient's temporomandibular joints and having him open and close his mouth a few times. The sensory functions of the nerve are tested by stimulation (e.g. with a pin or cotton wool) on the upper and lower jaw and around the eye, and the patient is asked to identify where he is touched each time. Normal trigeminal function serves the corneal reflex: as the person looks upward the doctor touches the cornea with a wisp of cotton and the eyelid normally closes.

VII Facial

The facial nerve has both motor and sensory functions. It controls the facial muscles and supplies taste fibres to the anterior two-thirds of the tongue.

Voluntary muscles of the face are tested by asking the patient to wrinkle his forehead and forcibly close his eyes, show his teeth, pucker his lips, whistle or smile. Asymmetrical movement, lack of mobility of facial expression or facial drooping are signs of disorder. Where a patient has peripheral facial paralysis, it becomes necessary to determine whether or not the taste fibres are involved.

Taste (*gustatory*) function is tested with sweet, sour and salt solutions on selected parts of the tongue. Lesions of the facial nerve are accompanied by impairment of taste on the front two-thirds of the tongue and lesions of the glossopharyngeal nerve by impairment on the posterior one-third.

VIII   Acoustic or Vestibulocochlear

The acoustic nerve controls both hearing and the sense of balance (*equilibrium*).

Hearing is tested with normal and whispered voice close to one ear while the other ear is blocked. Neural disorder is indicated if the patient cannot hear even when the eardrum is bypassed by placing the stem of a vibrating tuning fork on the mastoid bone behind the ear. For a more precise examination the patient attends the clinic for an audiometry test.

The vestibular portion of the nerve is tested by the 'past-pointing' test. The patient is asked to raise his arm and to bring the index finger down on the examiner's finger with the patient's arm outstretched, first with the eyes open, then with them closed. In vestibular disease the finger past-points to one side or the other consistently.

IX   Glossopharyngeal   X   Vagus

The glossopharyngeal and vagus nerves control swallowing, the gag reflex, articulation and phonation.

The glossopharyngeal is tested by observing the movement and sensibility of the pharynx during examination of the mouth and throat. The larynx may be tested by studying the timbre of the voice, and where the patient has hoarseness or aphonia a laryngoscopic examination will be made.

The taste function is assessed during examination for the facial nerve. Some impairment of the vagus nerve is present if the patient has difficulty in talking and swallowing. Paralysis on one side is indicated by movement of the palate to the opposite side.

XI   Spinal accessory

The spinal accessory nerve controls the trapezius and sternocleidomastoid muscles. These muscles assist the patient in shoulder shrugging and head and neck movements. To assess trapezius muscle function the patient is asked to raise both shoulders against resistance. To test the opposite sternocleidomastoid muscle the patient is instructed to rotate his head against resistance applied to the side of the chin. Both sternocleidomastoids may be tested simultaneously by flexing the head forward against resistance under the chin.

XII   Hypoglossal

The hypoglossal nerve controls tongue movement and strength. This function is appraised by having the patient stick out his tongue, which normally protrudes in the mid-line. A tendency to protrude the tongue to one side indicates weakness of muscles in that half of the tongue. Tongue strength is tested by instructing the patient to move his tongue to the right and left. The examiner will be particularly alert for signs of trembling (*fibrillation*) or other unusual movements.

The motor system

The cerebral cortex of the brain is composed of many layers of nerve cells arranged in irregular folds and convolutions. In front of one of these folds, the central sulcus or Fissure of Rolando, there are thousands of motor nerve cells. These are large, pyramid-shaped cells that form the beginning of the motor pathway that controls movement of the body. Voluntary motor function is controlled mainly by the pyramidal tracts, which descend through the brain stem, the tracts from the left side of the brain crossing to the right side and those from the right side crossing to the left. Awareness of these physiological facts enables nurses to explain to the patient why the doctor has to examine both sides of his body in order to observe any abnormalities, why a problem that he has been told is on the left side of his brain is causing right-sided symptoms.

Damage to motor cells and fibres produces muscle weakness, muscle wasting and alterations in muscle tone (the degree of tension felt in a muscle at rest). The degree of tone influences the behaviour of the tendon reflexes. Depending on where the lesion is in the motor system, the patient will experience slight or very marked wasting and weakness and increased or decreased tone. Observations of changes in reflexes and involuntary movements also enable the doctor to put all the evidence together to reach a diagnosis.

Examining the motor system

Examination of the motor system includes determination of muscle power, bulk and tone, observation of the occurrence of involuntary muscle movements, and assessment of the status of the reflexes.

Muscle size

Comparison of the same muscle on either side of the body is made by palpation for wasting or atrophy. Muscle bulk can be measured with a tape measure if there is a question of difference in size. Abnormalities could include *atrophy* (wasting of muscle tissue) or *hypertrophy* (excessive thickening of muscle tissue).

Muscle tone

The tone of each muscle is systematically assessed at rest and during a passive range of motion, and both sides of the body are compared to determine equality or inequality. Included in the assessment are the muscles of the neck, back, shoulders, arms, legs and hips. Abnormalities could include *spasticity* (increased tone of muscle tissue, rigidity) or *flaccidity* (loss of muscle tone, floppiness).

Muscle strength

Muscles of the major joints are put through the normal range of motion, first against gravity, then against active resistance; comparison of the same muscles on each side of the body is made to note strength or weakness. The hand grip is tested by asking the patient to squeeze the examiner's fingers. The power of the hand grip is determined by the force required to withdraw the fingers. Power in the arms is tested by asking the patient to flex and extend the forearm against resistance. When the patient has a history of specific neck, shoulder or arm pain, the shoulder girdle muscles will be examined particularly carefully. The legs are also tested by asking the patient to flex and extend them against resistance. Doctors and physiotherapists whose daily activity entails muscle testing make it look very easy, but nurses using these tests should seek advice on the correct methods of holding arms and joints to avoid forcing spastic limbs to conform to a neurological observations chart.

Involuntary movements

1. *Tremors:* involuntary trembling of any part of the body.
2. *Tics:* involuntary twitchings of a muscle.
3. *Myoclonus:* sudden, brief jerking contraction of a muscle or muscle group.
4. *Athetosis:* slow, writhing movements of a limb, the trunk or face.
5. *Choreiform movements:* irregular, jerky uncoordinated movements and abnormal posture.
6. *Fasiculations:* isolated fine twitches of muscle fibres due to contraction of a single motor unit, which can be seen and felt through the skin.

(See also Chapter 2, 'Involuntary movements', Chapter 3, 'Movement disorders'.)

The sensory system

Sensory nerve impulses travel in ascending tracts. These afferent impulses are interpreted by the sensory area of the cerebral cortex so that the various modalities of sensation, e.g. touch, pain, itch, temperature and warm and cold sensations, can be appreciated. The sensory fibres in the peripheral nerves and spinal cord carry a constant flow of information about the postural arrangement of the patient's limbs and joints.

Patients generally do not report a loss of sensation, at least not in those terms. They often say that a part feels numb or dead or that it has a funny feeling. Clumsiness of movement may be a reflection of a loss of spatial sense. The patient may compensate for this loss by carefully watching his movements, so it is necessary to have the patient close his eyes when dexterity of movement is being tested. Walking can be tested by getting the patient to walk in a straight line with the eyes closed. However, if he tends to fall, it is important for him to know that the nurse is there beside him during the test: 'I won't let you fall' is a necessary reassurance that can be offered.

Sensation is normally well appreciated over the body surface and felt equally over both sides of the body, limbs and face. When a person has sensory impairment, it becomes necessary to investigate the degree of sensory loss and the distribution of this loss. There are different degrees of sensory impairment and the nurse who understands the terminology can help the patient who worries about long words used by the doctor:

- Complete sensory loss – *anaesthesia* (touch); *analgesia* (pain);
- Partial sensory loss – *hypalgesia*;
- An increase of feeling on stimulation – *hyperaesthesia*;
- Spontaneous feelings without stimulation – *paraesthesia*;
- Clumsiness of movement, including unsteadiness of gait.

(See Chapter 5, 'Ronald'.)

Sensation is usually tested at the end of the examination, which should not be too lengthy as fatigue sets in rapidly and replies become increasingly inaccurate. The three main questions to be considered are: what elements of sensation are affected; how widespread is the involvement: and where is the sensory loss? The same areas on opposite sides of the body are assessed and compared for the various sensory perceptions.

Evaluation

Superficial (light) touch is tested using a piece of cotton wool. It should be a light touch and not a tickle. All areas of the skin of the trunk, extremities and face are tested, and a comparison is made of the intensity of the stimuli needed for a response in various areas. Superficial pain sensitivity of the skin is tested by light pricking with a pin and the ability of the patient to localise the exact place just pricked (without having looked). Temperature sensation is tested by the application of hot and cold water tubes to the skin. Comparison of the ability to recognise differences between hot and cold stimuli is made for all parts of the body. The sensing of changes in the muscles and joints (*proprioception*) is indicated by the ability to recognise passive movements of the joints and detect vibrations produced by a tuning fork on the body prominences and on the skin.

Balance

Normal balance is the result of a number of different functions that combine to achieve an integrated, although constantly changing, sensory pattern. If a person has balance problems so that he tends to fall over, gets dizzy spells or cannot walk with ease, there are many different causes and different places in the body where these may lie. Many neurological disorders are evident in the patient's gait, indicating possible disturbances of cerebellar function that may result in defects of coordination, balance, speech, eyes, neck, trunk and limb movement. The clinical examination may, therefore, devote more time to evaluation of balance than is usually seen in a general medical examination. The patient will need plenty of room as he will be asked to walk briskly with his eyes open and closed and to turn quickly. He will be asked to perform the complex activities requiring coordination that are described below, and most people are happier if the nurse can explain some of these tests in advance, as this makes for a more relaxed atmosphere in the consulting room. (See also Chapter 2, 'Dizziness and vertigo'.)

Examination

In the finger–nose test, the patient is asked to touch the doctor's moving index finger and then his own nose. The test may be varied by asking the patient to touch his nose in rapid succession several times. This is normally performed smoothly and easily with eyes both open and closed. For the Romberg test the patient stands with his feet together and arms at his sides, with his eyes first open and then closed. The test is considered positive only if there is an actual loss of balance after 10 seconds. The nurse should stand close to the patient (to catch him if he falls) but not touch him. The patient may be asked to walk as if he is measuring the floor with the heel of one foot placed against the front of the toe of the other with each step. It is impossible for patients with cerebellar dysfunction to perform this tandem walking test.

For the heel–knee test the patient lies in the supine position with the heel of one foot placed on the opposite knee. This should be done smoothly, without tremor and with accuracy. The foot may then be slid down the shin, again a movement performed smoothly and evenly in people who do not have a balance problem. To discover the strength and coordination of the muscles on one side of the body and determine minimal motor disorder, the patient is requested to hop continuously, first on one foot and then on the other (the nurse should be ready to assist if the patient falters). Any inequality in performance of the hopping test will be followed by more careful assessment of leg strength, tone and coordination.

The reflexes

The reflex arc is the simplest functional unit of the nervous system capable of detecting change and causing a response to that change. Many body activities are controlled reflexly. This term implies an automatic adjustment to maintain homeostasis without conscious effort. Reflex activity is involuntary but can often be stopped by an act of will; if we expect a certain stimulus we need not respond to it. Reflex activity is stereotyped so that stimulation of a given receptor always causes the same effector response. Thus, if the patella tendon is tapped, the knee always extends: it is therefore predictable. Sometimes the patient will be asked to pull on his clenched hands at the moment his patella is tapped in order to reinforce the response. When a muscle is stretched, nerve impulses from a muscle spindle pass into the spinal cord and act on the anterior horn cells that supply the adjacent motor units. The anterior horn cells send nerve impulses along the motor nerves and the motor units contract: the *stretch reflex*. The pathway is termed a *monosynaptic reflex arc* since only one synapse is involved.

Stretch reflexes are found in all the muscles of the body. If any muscle is stretched it will promptly contract. It is technically difficult to stretch some muscles, but in certain parts of the body muscles can be stretched easily. The quadriceps muscle of the thigh has a tendon that passes round the lower end of the femur and is inserted into the tibia. Embedded in the middle of this tendon is a short sessamoid bone known as the patella. Tiny sessamoid bones in tendons at points of friction are also found in the interphalangeal and metacarpophalangeal joints. By tapping the tendon between the patella and the tibia with a rubber-covered patella hammer, a pull is exerted on the quadriceps muscle. The monosynaptic reflex causes the muscle to contract. The resultant contraction extends the knee and kicks the foot forward in the knee jerk. When neurological disease interferes with the reflex arc itself, this is seen in decreased tendon reflexes, as in diseases of the peripheral nerves. Reflexes may be increased when the patient has had a cerebrovascular accident or has motor neurone disease affecting the upper motor neurones that would normally inhibit the reflex arc to facilitate organised movement.

Testing reflexes

To test deep tendon reflexes (biceps and triceps reflexes) the tendon of the joint is tapped, which normally results in the contraction of the muscle and a quick movement of the extremity. Tendon reflexes in the extremities are elicited by placing a finger on the tendon (just below the kneecap) and tapping the tendon briskly with a soft hammer.

Superficial reflexes are elicited by a light, rapid stroking of the skin or mucous membrane in a particular area, such as the superficial abdominal reflexes. The Babinski reflex is the most important: an orange stick is stroked across the lateral aspect of the patient's sole from the heel to the ball of the foot; the response is positive when the hallux (big toe) goes up, with fanning of the other toes.

Abnormal reflexes

Abnormal responses of deep tendon reflexes are either *hypereflexic*, an exaggerated reflex response, or *hyporeflexic*, a diminished reflex response to stimuli.

Superficial reflexes should not appear in the normally healthy person. The grasp reflex occurs when the stimulus of stroking the palm of the patient's hand is followed by the patient grasping the examiner's fingers between his thumb and index finger and holding on against resistance. Two reflexes that are normal in infancy, but if present in the adult indicate some neurological deficit, are the sucking reflex when an object comes in contact with the lips, and the Babinski reflex (described above).

The abdominal reflex is lost in upper motor neurone lesions such as cerebrovascular accident and they may be difficult to elicit in the elderly, in the obese and in women whose abdominal muscles are stretched after childbirth. In adults the Babinski response is abnormal and is seen in upper motor neurone lesions and in the early stages of a cerebrovascular accident when the patient is comatose and tone and reflexes have not yet increased. This is very similar to the infantile response when the great toe is dorsiflexed and the other toes extend and fan out.

Conclusion of the clinical examination

At the end of the clinical examination the doctor will discuss his observations and conclusions with the patient and any accompanying relatives or friends whom the patient wishes to participate in the consultation. The doctor will also offer advice on further investigations and plans for the future. The patient may be asked if he is willing to have specific tests: because each person's problems are assessed individually, it is usually impossible to be able to tell patients in advance what tests and treatment they are likely to require.

The diagnosis

Neurological disorders

Myths

1. Most people have heard of Parkinson's disease, but their knowledge of the condition usually dates from the period before modern treatment became available. Patients blame their disease on some traumatic experience: an injury, illness or surgical operation. Overindulgence in alcohol, tobacco, tea or coffee, having a weight problem or being lazy are all mythical notions about the cause of Parkinson's disease and are totally unsupported by facts.
2. Multiple sclerosis is often associated with a tragedy that afflicts a talented young person, who will inevitably become a wheelchair 'cabbage' with an early death. Such gloom may raise funds for charities, but it hangs 'like an albatross' over the heads of newly diagnosed patients. In itself, this is disabling, regardless of the presence or absence of symptoms.
3. People with hearing disorders are treated as though they have intellectual damage, rather than a sensory loss.
4. Having an epileptic disorder means that the person has to adjust to a society that clings to ancient stigmatising associations about 'epileptics', with connotations of madness and 'sins of the fathers'.
5. The presence of a tremor or other involuntary movement makes observers think the victim is 'crazy' or has had too much to drink.
6. The families of some people with Huntington's chorea have been scorned and ridiculed because the sufferers were suspected of drug or alcohol abuse by an uninformed public. Until friends or neighbours make some comment about alcohol, a person may be unaware that when he walks he sways about.

Facts

1. There are very few predictable disease processes in neurology – each patient's experience of a disorder is unique.
2. Most disorders of the nervous system, e.g. epileptic seizure, migraine, vertigo or tremor attack, result in impaired function, at least while the disorder is being experienced.
3. Talking about a degenerative disease can have severe emotional overtones. It can only be conveyed successfully to the patient and family members in an atmosphere of empathy, warmth and understanding.
4. Medical and psychosocial needs are interrelated and are a vital part of the patient's and family's adjustment.
5. Out-of-date books may only provide depressing advice that takes no account of recent developments in treatment.
6. Reactions of the patient who knows his neurological diagnosis vary from unrealistic expectations of a cure to deep depression and the temptation to commit suicide.

The undiagnosed condition

When the presence of a disease or condition is not demonstrated through a classic series of signs and symptoms, the patient's complaints are easily thought to be caused by tiredness, overwork or hypochondria – this causes considerable confusion to patient and family alike. The longer a condition is allowed to continue undiagnosed the harder it is for patients to convince their families that they have a real dysfunction and need support and help.

The diagnosis of multiple sclerosis is difficult in the early stages. It is often suspected when the clinical evidence is still insufficient to make the diagnosis more than a possibility: there is no specific laboratory test and a firm diagnosis cannot be given where doubt exists. Diagnostic difficulties can arise if the symptoms are vague, transient or poorly defined – they can resemble the symptoms of anxiety or depression and may be dismissed by the doctor as unimportant, or as a reason for prescribing tranquillisers or antidepressant drugs. Symptoms of this sort include fatigue, dizzy spells, strange sensations, pins and needles, difficulty in concentrating and loss of memory.

In those families who know of the risk of Huntington's chorea, it is often a close relative who detects the first signs, especially when these appear as subtle changes of mood and personality. There is no predictive test and the doctor may only reach a diagnosis when several aspects of the disease, i.e. intellectual impairment, involuntary movement and a positive family history, are present. The confusing pattern that delays or hinders a correct diagnosis means that the psychological problems caused by the disease may be confused with psychiatric illness.

One significant problem associated with Alzheimer's disease is that of diagnosis itself. Not only does the disease exist in two forms – early and late – but the symptoms are also easily confused with the reversible loss of memory and other intellectual functions that may be caused by depression, drugs and metabolic and endocrine disturbances.

The average doctor will only see one or two patients with myasthenia gravis during his career. Scadding and Havard (1981) say that 'A diagnosis of psychiatric illness is commonly made'. A young nurse who has difficulty lifting patients may be medically diagnosed as hysterical but her muscle weakness may later be identified as myasthenic.

Many adults with Gilles de la Tourette syndrome had their condition wrongly diagnosed during childhood, so they can become disenchanted with the medical profession and reluctant to attend even a single hospital appointment. Some patients have spent considerable periods of time in psychiatric institutions and received a wide variety of treatments that will not have helped their condition (Lees et al, 1984).

Needing a name

A great deal of conflict sometimes arises between patients and physicians during the period before a neurological diagnosis is made. Many patients begin to take an active part in discovering their own diagnosis and these conflicts can extend to relationships with family and friends. However, 'naming the disease' can, strangely enough, lead to a reduction of stress. Often people with, for example, multiple sclerosis speak of relief at knowing their diagnosis; naturally, many are shocked and distressed, but at least they know the truth and can begin to come to terms with it – the truth is rarely worse than the unknown.

Knowing the diagnosis helps to make the illness more tolerable than a nameless fear. Patients tend to explain that they were almost relieved when they knew the worst; they felt calmer and better able to cooperate with the health-care professionals trying to help them. The patient has to be able to understand the changes that are occurring in his body.

The diagnosed patient

'Telling the truth' to the patient and relatives is basically a counselling exercise requiring an understanding of psychological processes, self-awareness and relationship skills, but the doctor does not always have sufficient time or the required training to do this properly. A nurse will often be able to help on these occasions and may be in a better position to provide the regular patient contact that is so necessary with neurological disorders. Opportunities must be provided for the patient and his relatives to return for more information and support, for it takes time for people to work through their feelings of shock, fear, anger and sadness at each stage of the disease. There must, therefore, be a shared understanding of each other's roles by all involved, as well as mutual trust and respect.

Facts alone are often insufficient, even if they are retained by the hearer. Several studies have shown that there is no relationship between knowledge about the condition or treatment recommendations and the person's success in following those recommendations. Distressed people listen and remember selectively: something told does not mean something heard and remembered. Checking what a person thinks he has been told and repeating corrected versions should be a routine, and information given needs to be realistic. Experience and research findings show that individuals and families respond best to explanations and offers of support while the condition is being diagnosed; this is at a time when they can both comprehend the explanation and utilise the help being offered.

The problem of how to answer the question — What is epilepsy, multiple sclerosis, etc.? — is related to and developed from an analysis of the needs of the family, the problems that they may encounter, their actual experience of the condition to be discussed and the likelihood of resources and referrals being available to assist at the time of particular need. Children can be very sensitive to anxiety and may become disruptive and attention-seeking if they are ignored. Facts should be explained to them and if they are involved in major family decisions, they will not feel excluded and resentful.

When families ask about a known diagnosis they are often concerned primarily with the psychosocial implications of the disorder and less with the medical aspects; the nurse is therefore an appropriate person to help the patient, provided she knows what these implications are and the need to base the answer on an understanding of the knowledge, attitudes and beliefs of the questioner.

When communicating with the patient at the time of diagnosis nurses and doctors should generate an atmosphere in which the patient and family can express their feelings about the diagnosis. Patients and family members have to be given a chance to evaluate the situation realistically in order to make plans for adjustment.

Having acknowledged the negative aspects of a disorder, the nurse has to emphasise what the patient *can* do, as the stress now has to be put on positive skills and strengths rather than on the negative.

It is important for the nurse to explain how the treatment programme will be designed. This will make things easier for the patient and his family or friends who may be closely involved with his experiences.

The patient may reject the diagnosis and seek other opinions, perhaps followed by investigations to exclude other disorders. He may accept the diagnosis and reject the doctor and everyone else working with him, concluding that as there is no specific therapy and as the course is unpredictable medical supervision has little to offer. Patients, relatives and close friends all need to be given the opportunity to 'work through' the feelings of shock, anger and resentment. Eventually they will reach a stage of acceptance when they can begin to get on with the business of everyday living.

Listening to the patient

The main object of talking is to get the patient to talk, to hear what he has to say, to listen and just to say enough to keep him talking. When a person knows that he has a good listener to talk to, he will share his thoughts more fully, which in turn makes it easier to help him with his problems. Hayward (1975) has found that nurses can lessen anxiety and therefore reduce pain by listening, by explanation and by recognising that the patient and his relatives are worried and need help. A good listener may help the patient psychologically by making him feel important enough for someone to listen to him or by relieving some of his inner tensions when he can talk out some of his thoughts.

When listening, one should do nothing else, not even think while listening, just let it sink in. Start where the patient starts and go along with him; only keep him moving from area to area, and move at his own pace if possible, until the feeling of knowing him comes. Try to be at home or relatively relaxed when talking or listening to a patient – the over-tense helper tends to leap in too quickly with a response every time he pauses.

Patients' attitudes

We tend to underestimate the level of understanding that patients are capable of achieving. Each patient has a positive part to play in his illness and contains within himself a potential for adjustment and finding satisfactory goals that will lead to a full satisfying life. Worry and anxiety can be related to lack of knowledge and not to the seriousness of the disease. Providing information will reduce the patient's fearful fantasies and thus help him to prepare for events that need to be recognised and accepted as normal.

The first steps are to assess and observe where the patient is in the long process of reacting to living with a progressive disorder, by placing oneself at the same point at which he is in understanding his symptoms. How much information will he need to be able to cope with his problems? How does he define his problems? What does he see as his main problem? How does he understand his symptoms? What are his fears? Sometimes the nurse has to think about a patient's questions in more depth, asking herself what lies behind the question and what made the patient ask it. What does the patient want to express? No magic rules are offered to the nurse who has to learn to differentiate between the request for factual information and expressed psychological needs. Nurses who are also parents will have already developed communication skills that others have to learn through nurse–patient relationships and participating in formal communication study days or workshops.

Patients' vocabulary

When a nurse asks a patient what his main problem is, she has to remember that specific medical terms often have quite different meanings to the patient. Some discussion of meanings may be necessary to reach common understanding of such terms as dizziness, faintness, blackout, double vision, spasm and numbness. Dizziness may be the term used to describe vertigo, syncope, unsteadiness or confusion. When a patient says that he cannot use his leg or arm, he may then go on to explain that this means that his legs are feeling stiff, tight or useless, i.e. spastic. Slow, painful, stiff or useless fingers that cannot do up buttons may indicate that he is suffering from rigidity or *akinesia*.

Complaints of feeling clumsy, weak or quickly tired, or always dropping things and feeling unsteady, may indicate the presence of *ataxia* (poor coordination). When the patient reports that his fingers feel numb and useless and that he has lost the ability to tell the temperature of water, this is a sign of a loss of superficial sensation. Patients often say that they are unsteady or numb when they mean weak. Other terms that could cause confusion include 'feeling sick', 'dizziness' or 'being nervous'. It is essential to ask the patient to elaborate on the terms he uses, particularly if the nurse is recording observations for use by colleagues in hospital or clinic.

Defining pain

How pain is described is influenced by a number of factors, including language facility, familiarity with medical terms, individual experiences of pain and lay beliefs about the structure and function of the body. The use of medical terms by a patient may confuse the doctor as, for example, when a patient says, 'I've had another migraine': he may be using the term to describe a wide variety of head pains, not only migraine. Medical history-taking, examinations and diagnostic tests may all train patients to identify and describe the characteristic form of a particular type of pain such as 'angina', 'colic' or 'migraine'.

The nurse can never know precisely what the patient is feeling. Pain is, therefore, a very complex phenomenon, which requires assessment if attempts at appropriate intervention are to be carried out. The simplest and most reliable index of pain is the patient's verbal report – words such as 'sharp', 'dull' and 'aching' may aid the nurse in assessing his pain and perhaps in determining its origin.

Anxious patients' questions

1. Does this mean I'm going 'mad'? Is it all in my mind, 'psychological'? Does frothing at the mouth in an epileptic seizure mean you're mad?
2. Is the disease caused by stress or shock?
3. Can people deliberately bring on seizures themselves?
4. Should I tell my employer/friends about this problem?

People who worry as in (1) may have suffered pain for a long time. Therefore, when all investigations have indicated negative results, they begin to doubt their own sanity because no one acknowledges the reality of their pain. Other patients who admit to having this worry similarly lack a diagnostic label: when the specialist does not know what is wrong with you, you begin to doubt yourself and wonder about your sanity.

The old historical notions of epilepsy and 'madness' create much suffering for individuals and their relatives when learning to live with an epileptic disorder. If we consider these worrying questions before they are put to us by anxious patients, our response will be more thoughtful than when confronted with them 'cold'.

Worries about the 'causes' of illnesses may be driven by a need to 'put the blame' on someone or something, because things seem more tolerable if they can be explained by a concrete event, i.e. an accident or infectious agent. Questions about voluntary will may occur more in the epilepsies than with other manifestations of disease, possibly because of the fears aroused in onlookers, which can be more vivid than seeing someone with a tremor or in a wheelchair. Trying to understand the fear behind questions is an important skill in nurse–patient interaction. Whether or not to tell one's employer about an epileptic disorder is controversial because honesty may lead to unemployment!

Non-verbal communication

A high proportion of interpersonal communication is through non-verbal behaviour. Most individuals trust the non-verbal messages they receive because they have learned that although people can lie verbally, it is hard to hide the lie when speaking. When verbal and non-verbal cues tell different stories, the non-verbal story tends to be believed. Words can be chosen with care but expressive non-verbal cues cannot be chosen. The body is not so easily governed. It is known that patients can become anxious when the non-verbal messages given by the staff (e.g. bustling behaviour) do not accord with what they are being told. Non-verbal features of communication are complex: they are used not only to complement the verbal features but also to convey messages of their own accord.

Actions not only speak louder than words but sometimes can also do instead of words: touch, movement, gestures and looks are communication methods that we all use unconsciously and can learn to use deliberately with great effect. Because of the degree of facial muscular development we are able to do many things with our faces. A patient may smile and say, 'I am all right', while in fact experiencing pain that is nothing to smile about, so as not to be a nuisance to the nurses. Thus, facial expression can reinforce the spoken words or wipe them out completely. Being aware of how the patient feels, and showing this understanding by facial expression and verbally, is known as empathy. Touch is the most personal of our senses in that it brings two human beings into close relationship. A touch coming at the right moment showing understanding, encouragement or compassion can communicate, to a patient or relative, more comfort than the giver may be aware of.

Losses

Patients seldom talk about their anxieties, even when asked. Nevertheless those who ask many questions, or who never ask at all, may be masking real anxiety. Individuals who are undecided keep asking different people for advice, obtaining contradictory views and continuing until they obtain an opinion that supports their own preference. If the patient is encouraged to talk about the expected consequences of changing his life-style, he will in the end be able to find ways of making adjustments to suit his needs.

Not all nurses are good conversationalists, good listeners or at ease in company. For many patients this does not matter because they have adequate resources in themselves, their families and friends and so do not have to rely on the nurse's social skills. Some patients do not seem to want nurses to talk to them at all and their wish to be left alone must be respected. There are, however, occasions when a patient's comments or questions are indications that it is appropriate for the nurse to respond carefully to his expressed psychological needs. The role of nursing is demonstrated by warm, unconditional acceptance of an individual.

Patients' questions – causes

What is the cause of my symptoms?   Is it due to a brain tumour?
How did I get it?   Is it inherited?   Who gets it?
Is Parkinson's disease due to a virus/'nerves'/a stroke/an injury?
Can it be caused by environmental poisons, dietary deficiency or drugs?
Is it contagious?   Is epilepsy an allergy?   Will my next child get it?
Does smoking in pregnancy cause epilepsy?   Why does a stroke occur?
What is happening inside my body?   Is a fit the same thing as epilepsy?
What is an aura?   What are absences?
What happens in a migraine/epileptic attack?
Can epilepsy occur with high blood pressure?
Can a bang on the head cause epilepsy?   What is status epilepticus?
Can I do anything to prevent a fit happening?
What did I do to deserve this?   Am I to blame for my child's fits?

Reactions to loss

When a person discovers that he has a neurological disorder, a 'progressively deteriorating condition', this comes as a great shock. His reaction is in some ways like experiencing a bereavement: he has lost a well-loved part of himself and has to substitute an unwelcome identity as a 'disabled person' for it. Anyone in this situation needs to cry, to be angry and to curse God or his ancestors and to ask 'Why me'? The anger needs to be directed somewhere: sometimes people find something in themselves to blame – 'those tablets I took', 'that injury I had' and so on. Nursing and medical staff may be convenient scapegoats and may be rejected or treated unfairly, which can lead to strained or broken relationships requiring much patience, understanding and time to repair. If the individual is not allowed to experience this mourning, he is unlikely ever to become adjusted to his new identity. In caring for a person psychologically, the object is not to find the right thing to say, not to turn off emotion and solve problems instantly – it is to provide the best environment for anxieties, anger and grief to be expressed, shared and clarified.

In order to come to terms with loss, a process of grieving or mourning may have to be experienced in a similar manner to those who must mourn or grieve for the loss of loved ones. Only when such processes have been worked through can individuals cope with death or disability. A death of the normal body has occurred, but society does not provide established rituals as guidelines for this type of loss. Often this leaves family members in the situation of misunderstanding one another's needs for support. The grief response to a change in body function and/or shape is a very individual thing, so each person should be helped to find the mode of grieving that is most emotionally comfortable to him. One must emphasise, however, that there are disabled individuals who may neither grieve nor mourn nor pass through a series of adjustment stages.

The process of mourning begins to resolve as the person comes to acknowledge the limitations imposed by the disability that may require his dependence on others. This physical dependence must be separated from a sense of devaluation as a person. Each individual must begin to tolerate his altered body in order to fuse his emotional, cognitive and physical identities, expecting that others who wish to share his life will respond similarly.

A woman who had maintained her personal identity despite dramatic changes caused by a neurological condition explained that she had to integrate her illness into her life without letting it take over completely, to make it part of her experience, not part of her personality. To ignore it and concentrate only on the times when it was in remission would mean ignoring large parts of her life. She felt that if she were to wait until she would be 'better' to consider her life worthwhile she could wait forever because she knew that she might never be 'better' again.

Adjusting to the threatened identity as a sexually normal person involves a restating of lovability by the disabled person; someone who can once again view himself as lovable, desirable and sexually competent. If disabled people cannot have these feelings towards themselves, it is almost impossible for them to believe that others can find them attractive and desirable.

Questions about the future

Do I have to stop smoking?   Will I have to stop drinking alcohol?
Do I need a special diet?   Do I have to stop driving?
How much rest should I have?   Can I continue with my sports?
Will it affect my ability to work/my leisure activities?
Will the fits impair my memory?

Personality loss – dementia

Dementia is not merely a loss of intellect but a disintegration of the self. Self involves having an identity in space and time and being able to create order and direction in the outside world, from the simplest manipulations through to the most complex. Dementia is a dismantling of the human being, starting at the most organised and complex part and proceeding to the failure of the components of the central nervous system. Rather than being aware that one is losing the functions of a number of organs through illness, one's whole awareness is itself affected.

Many dementing patients are aware of their deterioration and some will even be able to describe it as mental sluggishness. With sluggishness comes sadness for the mental life they used to have, a memory of acuteness and mental ability, the sort of sadness that resembles grief for a dead relative. As in bereavement, grief can be coped with better if verbalised to an empathetic listener, so this sadness is helped by talking. A reminiscence of previous achievements will also aid the retention of dignity. (See also Chapter 4, 'Feelings'.)

Denial

Each person with a chronic neurological disorder undergoes a process of evaluating his continued physical existence that results in an active, conscious decision to live. Some people need to separate themselves mentally from their bodies while struggling to combat the lack of a sense of wholeness they are experiencing: this is a healthy coping mechanism by which to escape from a tortured body. With some types of disability it is possible to deny the long-term effects, but with others the changes are so total that withdrawal seems to be the only way to carry on. Others become enraged at God, their family, the situation or themselves. On a rational level, there is a search for a reason for the disability that requires an emotional response. For some people a sense of punishment or omen is the first in a series of emotional possibilities that they identify in this quest. People with a negative self-image who view themselves as being victims of fate see the disability as a symbol of their badness.

Some people need to deny part of the truth until they can cope with it all. Therefore, skill is needed to assess how much individuals really want to know at any one time. Denial of the symptoms of the disease can take many forms. Often, people will be unable to admit to themselves that they have a neurological disease and they need time to understand the implications before they can tell other people what their trouble really is. For this reason, families and employers are frequently excluded from knowing the true situation and may show little or no understanding.

Epilepsy

The tendency of people with an epileptic disorder to avoid disclosure of the information outside the family is a complicated subject. Nurses are required to consider several conflicting points of view and then to understand why this behaviour occurs with the individual concerned. There are many popular misconceptions about the effect of epilepsy on people's lives, especially their working lives, and people have been refused jobs when it became known that they had epilepsy. Someone with epilepsy may be feared because, without warning and in any situation, he may lose control of his movements. We are all afraid of losing control – making a fool of ourselves in public – and the person with epilepsy reminds us of this basic fear of reverting to the 'primitive', even losing control of the bladder in public. Every nurse can therefore understand the fears of the patient who has to live with the unpredictable nature of epileptic fits.

Multiple sclerosis

People will often resort to all sorts of alternative diets and treatments in order to try to find a cure for multiple sclerosis. This can be their way of refusing to accept reality, of pretending that multiple sclerosis is a curable disease. However, it can lead them to spend vast amounts of money in order to buy useless treatments that may even be dangerous. Coming to terms with multiple sclerosis is about finding the balance between, on the one hand, completely giving in to the disease and, on the other, completely denying it and refusing to accept it. Instead of finding a balance, some patients may initially react in the extreme before they find the middle path. It is the nurse's duty to her patient to communicate the fact that it is only a small minority of people with the disorder who become disabled. There are many people leading quite normal lives who have been diagnosed as having multiple sclerosis and who may spend years without experiencing any noticeable symptoms. The 'doom-and-gloom philosophy' is not constructive in communication with such people.

Huntington's chorea

Many individuals at risk of developing a genetic neurological disorder find that their spouses, their immediate family or their relatives are too involved, too frightened or too guilty really to listen to the genetic counsellor. Most people at risk do not wish to frighten their families with their concerns nor do they want other family members to watch them for symptoms. Because of their own difficulties in coping with the risk situation, family members often brush aside the concerns of the at-risk person. Spouses will deny the reality: 'Don't worry, I won't let you get it'. It means that the disease is truly too terrible to think about. Despite having a realistic appraisal of the situation, a conspiracy of silence regarding the disease can grow between a couple because each does not want to frighten the other (Wexler, 1979).

Example: A husband with a sense of loss
    A housewife who was exceptionally clever at preparing meals and making gateaux and who entertained frequently found that because of the onset of multiple sclerosis she could no longer continue with her normal activities. For her husband the biggest tragedy was the loss of her ability to concentrate – he felt a sense of loss because neither he nor their daughters had any communication whatsoever with her and he had to make all the decisions in the house. He got little sleep as he was up two or three times a night to take her to the lavatory. The presence of multiple sclerosis completely changed their life-style.

Example: Loss of the will to live
    A man with a 10-year history of myasthenia gravis was re-admitted to hospital as the result of a chest infection and had to be put on a ventilator. The nurses found that he was very depressed and seemed to have lost the will to live. Unfortunately, their observations were correct. Despite all their efforts to help him to regain his 'fight', he admitted that he no longer wanted to live because he was such a burden to his family. Had he been able to experience the anger and grief at the loss of his personal self-image, he would have

accepted his new 'disabled' identity and found a new purpose in life instead of giving up the struggle.

References

Blau J N (1984) Fears aroused in patients by migraine. *British Medical Journal,* **288**(1): 1126.

Greene J G, Smith R, Gardiner M and Timbury G C (1982) Measuring behavioural disturbance of elderly demented patients in the community and its effects on relatives: a factor analytic study. *Age and Ageing,* **11:** 121–126.

Hayward J (1975) *Information – A Prescription Against Pain.* London: Royal College of Nursing.

Helman C (1984) *Culture, Health and Illness.* Bristol: John Wright.

Hough A (1986) Handling the patient in pain. *Nursing Times,* **82**(15): 28–31.

Lees A J, Robertson M, Trimble M R and Murray N M F (1984) A clinical study of Gilles de la Tourette syndrome in the United Kingdom. *Journal of Neurology, Neurosurgery & Psychiatry,* **47:** 1–8.

Maybury C P and Brewin C R (1984) Social relationships, knowledge and adjustment to multiple sclerosis. *Journal of Neurology, Neurosurgery and Psychiatry,* **47**(4): 372–376.

Melzack R (1975) The McGill pain questionnaire: major properties and scoring methods. *Pain,* **1:** 277–299.

Newrick P G and Langton-Hewer R (1984) Motor neurone disease; can we do better? A study of 42 patients. *British Medical Journal,* **289**(2): 539–542.

Oxtoby M (1982) *Parkinson's Disease Patients and their Social Needs.* London: Parkinson's Disease Society.

Scadding G F and Havard C W H (1981) Pathogenesis and treatment of myasthenia gravis. *British Medical Journal,* **282**(2): 1008–1012.

Wexler N S (1979) Genetic 'Russian roulette'. The experience of being 'at risk' for Huntington's disease. In: *Genetic Counselling Psychological Dimensions,* ed. Kessler S, p. 217. London: Academic Press.

Further reading

Assessment

Holland N J, Francabandera F and Weisel-Levison P (1986) International scale for assessment of disability in multiple sclerosis. *Journal of Neuroscience Nursing,* **18**(1): 39–44.

Latham J (1986) Assessment, observations and measurement of pain. *Professional Nurse,* **1**(4): 107–110.

McCurren C A and Ganong L H (1984) Assessing cognitive functioning of the elderly with the 'inventory of Piaget's developmental tasks'. *Journal of Advanced Nursing,* **9**(5): 449–456.

Clinical examination

Allan D (1986) Raised intracranial pressure. *Professional Nurse,* **2**(3): 78–80.

Bickerton J and Small J C (1981) *Neurology for Nurses.* London: Heinemann.

Nathan P (1988) *The Nervous System,* 3rd edn. Oxford: Oxford University Press.

Craigmyle M B L (1985) *The Mixed Cranial Nerves.* Chichester: John Wiley and Sons.

Davis B (1982) Tell them like it is. *Nursing Mirror,* **154**(12): 26–82.

Kocen R S (1976) *The Neuromuscular System.* Edinburgh: Churchill Livingstone.

Liebman M (1979) *Neuroanatomy Made Easy and Understandable.* Baltimore: University Park Press.

Walleck C A (1982) A neurologic assessment procedure that won't make you nervous. *Nursing (USA),* **12**(12): 50–58.

Wyness M A (1985) Perceptual dysfunction: Nursing assessment and management. *Journal of Neurosurgical Nursing,* **17**(2): 105–110.

Diagnosis

Blumhardt L (1986) Fits, faints and funny turns. *The Practitioner*, **230**(1412): 117–122.

Mahendra B (1985) The diagnosis trap. *Nursing Times*, **81**(30): 25–26.

Listening

Argyle M (1969) *Social Interaction*. London: Tavistock.

Argyle M, Furnham A and Graham J A (1981) *Social Situations*. Cambridge: Cambridge University Press.

Argyle M and Henderson M (1985) *The Anatomy of Relationships: The Rules and Skills Needed to Manage Them Successfully*. London: Heinemann.

Bridge W and Macleod Clark J (1981) *Communication in Nursing Care*. London: HM+M.

Brown H and Stevens R (eds.) (1975) *Social Behaviour and Experience: Multiple Perspectives*. London: Hodder and Stoughton (in association with The Open University).

Burton G (1977) *Interpersonal Relations: A Guide for Nurses*. London: Tavistock.

Eastwood C (1985) Communication breakdown. *Senior Nurse* **2**(9): 20–22.

Eastwood C M (1985) The role of communication in nursing – perceptual variations in student/teacher responses in Northern Ireland. *Journal of Advanced Nursing*, **10**(3): 245–250.

Gahogan J (1984) *Social Interaction and its Management*. London: Methuen.

Hinde R A (ed.) (1972) *Non-Verbal Communication*. Cambridge: Cambridge University Press.

Kubler-Ross E (1975) *Death: The Final Stage of Growth*. New Jersey: Prentice-Hall.

Le Moy A (1986) The human connection. *Nursing Times*, **82**(47): 28–30.

McIntosh J (1977) *Communication and Awareness in a Cancer Ward*. London: Croom Helm.

McGillaway O and Myco F (1985) *Nursing and Spiritual Care*. London: Harper and Row.

Chapter 2

PROBLEMS EXPERIENCED BY PATIENTS

────────── **Chapter theme** ──────────

Factual information about the main difficulties with which the neurological patient has to cope is the focus of this chapter. On first meeting such a patient, ordinary social courtesies may be impossible because he is confused and disorientated or could have a speech or hearing disorder. Closer observation and involvement with the patient and his relatives permits the nurse to become aware of his episodes of rigidity, fatigue or dizziness. Ultimately, in a practical nursing situation she will be involved in alleviating his pain, overcoming his dysphagia or discussing the effects of disability on his sexual relationships.

It is tempting to assume that all patients who grimace and leap about are psychologically disturbed when, in fact, they may be suffering from one of a number of well-known neurological disorders described in the 'Involuntary movements' section of this chapter. Similarly, when a patient explains that he has no energy, it is important for the nurse to know that his fatigue is due to a neurological disorder and is not necessarily a sign of depression or low motivation.

It can be confusing to see a patient stride along one day and then on another occasion find him rigid and 'frozen to the spot'. The 'Rigidity and fatigue' section will help the nurse to recognise the disorders that produce these problems. When the patient talks to the nurse about his giddiness, it is important to recognise the semantic confusions that can arise by different uses of terminology. The 'Dizziness and vertigo' section also provides a brief discussion of the mechanism of balance and draws attention to some of the causes of vertigo.

A survey of what nurses know about headache would possibly reveal familiarity with post-myelogram, tension and migraine headaches, but few would have had time to study the differentiating features of these problems. The section on 'Pain' examines the psychological and cultural aspects of pain, with a reminder of the physical symptoms that can be observed. The notes differentiating the experience of different types of headache in patients who have migraine, cluster or tension headache should be of use to the nurse who wants to be consistent in her use of terminology.

The nurse's interest in talking about or helping the patient who has difficulty in feeding himself will be heightened if she can understand some of the causes discussed in the section on 'Dysphagia'.

Sexuality is an integral part of every human being and the nurse's concern for improving the quality of life for patients must consider this aspect of neurological disease, which is discussed in 'Sexuality' at the end of the chapter.

Contents

Dementia

A middle-aged or elderly patient with a vacant, bemused expression on his face comes to see the physician, accompanied by his wife, one of his children or a concerned-looking relative. When offered a particular chair he may choose to sit on another one and does not seem to comprehend what is being said to him. The patient appears physically normal; he says he is not ill and that the anxiety of his relatives is without basis. His problems will be related by his relative, and he has no knowledge of the reason for the medical consultation.

Definitions

Dementia is the term applied to a diffuse deterioration of mental function. This results from organic disease of the brain and manifests itself, primarily, in thought and memory and, secondarily, in feeling and conduct. It may be produced by a large number of pathological changes, its effect varying according to the previous temperament of the patient, the age of onset, and the localisation, rate of progress and nature of the causal disorder (Walton, 1977).

Short-term memory is affected the most in dementia; there is an inability to memorise or store new knowledge and thus an inability to recall recent experiences. Long-term memory is the retrieval of older memories, particularly those formed before the onset of dementia. It is usually less affected, meaning that the person literally lives in the past because he cannot live in the present. However, the process of getting past events into the right order is often disrupted.

The patient becomes careless of his personal condition and fails to cope with the everyday tasks of sustaining life and an independent existence. He has wide mood swings, with emotional outbursts often alien to his character, and is given to morbid rumination. Usually memory, learning, orientation and conceptual thought are impaired. Poor intellectual grasp, poor memory and specific disabilities cause disorientation in three ways: getting lost in space and time, losing a sense of familiarity with the environment and becoming unaware of the progress of events in the outside world.

Causes

Alzheimer's disease
cerebrovascular disease, e.g.
   multi-infarct dementia
metabolic and deficiency states
alcoholism
Huntington's chorea

normal pressure hydrocephalus
Wilson's disease
syphilis
drug toxicity
intracranial tumour
Parkinson's disease

Alzheimer's disease

Alzheimer's disease is the most likely cause of dementia in a person more than 40 years old. There is a diffuse degeneration of the cerebral cortex, involving all its layers but most marked in the frontal lobes. Frontal lobe involvement can cause incontinence and a slow shuffling gait, which accompanies the intellectual deterioration. As the disease progresses there is complete disorientation. The duration of the disease is from $1\frac{1}{2}$ to 15 years (Harding, 1985). (See Chapter 3, 'Dementing disorders'.)

Cerebral atherosclerosis

Diffuse cerebrovascular disease is probably the second most common cause of dementia (Harding, 1985). Repeated episodes of cerebral infarction, producing areas of softening, may give rise to progressive impairment of memory and intellectual function. This is often accompanied by epileptic attacks and, ultimately, leads to an irreversible dementia with incontinence.

Intracranial tumour

Dementia can be caused by a primary or secondary intracranial tumour, involving particularly the frontal lobes. Memory and intellect can be severely affected while other aspects of behaviour and personality are reasonably well preserved. If the patient also has headaches and vomiting, these, combined with papilloedema, indicate raised intracranial pressure. In the most severely affected patient, intellectual capacity deteriorates so that he becomes stupid; he fails to appreciate the gravity of his illness, is careless of his dress and appearance and develops incontinence of urine and faeces without exhibiting any sense of impropriety. Such patients are sometimes jocular and facetious and repeatedly make simple jokes or puns. Irritability of temper and depression are not uncommon.

Cerebrospinal fluid

Normal pressure hydrocephalus is a condition in which normal circulation and reabsorption of cerebrospinal fluid are impaired as a result of subarachnoid haemorrhages or meningitis. The patient suffers from dementia, difficulty in walking (a gait disturbance) and incontinence of faeces and urine. Dementia due to normal pressure hydrocephalus begins during middle life. This is the only form of dementia in which relieving the peak cerebrospinal fluid (CSF) pressures, via a valve following a shunt operation, can produce marked improvement.

Acquired immune deficiency syndrome (AIDS)

The acquired immune deficiency syndrome is a new and epidemic form of profound cellular immunodeficiency, which is caused by a retrovirus known as HTLV-III. It acts on the body's cellular immune system, causing a depletion of the special T_4-helper cells that stimulate cellular immunity in the presence of an antigen. This allows the suppressor cells to multiply and to suppress cellular immunity when an antigen is absent. As a result of this, the immune response is very limited and the body is prone to opportunistic infections. The virus is transmitted through sexual intercourse, parenterally or perinatally.

The consequences of this infection on the nervous system are twofold. First, the immunodeficiency leads to a particular group of secondary or opportunist infections. Second, the HTLV-III retrovirus directly infects brain tissue. Secondary infections of the CNS include cryptococcal and tuberculous meningitis, toxoplasma abscesses, encephalitis and, less often, fungal abscesses. Cerebral lymphoma in isolation or as part of more widespread B-cell lymphoma is the only tumour to affect the CNS in AIDS. The direct infection of the nervous system causes a progressive dementia, which commences with personality changes and memory disturbance and leads to the most heartbreaking aspect of the AIDS syndrome – the patient becomes demented (Pinching, 1986).

Social consequences

Most elderly demented people live at home: some are able to rely on relatives and friends for support while others have to fend for themselves. The loss of communication skills inherent in dementia greatly impedes the ability to maintain or replace social contacts. Eventually this results in a progressively isolated existence, which lacks both internal and external sources of stimulation.

One of the most upsetting aspects of dementia is the impact that it has on the person's ability to communicate: his attention wanders, he may make illogical remarks, may not appear to hear or be influenced by what other people say or may repeat himself. These inappropriate responses are partly due to his dementing condition and partly caused or aggravated by the way in which other people speak to him. The nurse may find that by holding the old person's hand while talking to him she can engage his attention more effectively and at the same time give him the comfort and communication of physical contact. During a home visit distracting background noise can be reduced by switching off the television and radio. It is necessary to give more information than one would to someone who does not have dementia, for instance by saying, 'The librarian will bring books to you at home in a few days' time' rather than, 'The housebound library service will visit soon'. Mistakes should be corrected as they are made but if the patient keeps making the same mistake, the nurse should try to distract him and his train of thought by walking with him to another room or by doing something different, such as playing a game of cards.

A diminishing ability to cope with everyday tasks generates a heavy dependence on the home care services. While a community-based service can effectively reduce the frequency of admission to hospital, this is only achieved at the expense of imposing a considerable burden on the relatives of some patients. Some families carry a considerable load even before they attend hospital to see a specialist consultant about their problems (Sanford, 1975).

Caring at home (Table 2.1)

Sleep disturbance was the problem most frequently encountered and was one of those most poorly tolerated by the carer. Urinary incontinence occurred in many patients and could be tolerated. However carers were not prepared to endure faecal incontinence in their dependants. Dangerous and irresponsible behaviour can threaten disaster to the patient and others, but supporters are able to contain it by practical measures such as turning off gas supplies at source and locking outside doors. Anxiety and/or depression has been observed in over 50 per cent of people caring for a dependent demented relative. Restriction of social life has often been noted. Many carers do not have a holiday for a considerable period of time and others feel unable to leave their dependant for more than an hour, so that activity outside the home is denied. A 'sitting service', 'respite' accommodation and relatives' support groups are all desperately needed to relieve the burden imposed on families with a dementing family member.

Although it may not seem to matter to a confused person whether it is day or night, a routine is in fact of great importance in helping the affected person to remain calm and happy. Regular times for waking, rising, meals and going to bed are all helpful and the old person should be told the time as often as possible. The development of a regular rhythm will do much to prevent sleeping problems and broken nights. An early start to the day, some physical exercise and a regular evening ritual are more effective than sleeping pills. The routine in the evening should follow the same pattern – a meal, some entertainment, a quiet time and a hot drink. This pattern, kept to the same times each evening, will, with a warm bed, promote sleep. It is also useful to encourage the old person to empty his bladder last thing before retiring. Exercise, both mental and physical, is important: a walk outside every day is very helpful, not only in keeping the old person fit but also in providing stimulation, promoting sleep and preventing nocturnal 'wandering'.

Table 2.1 *Problems encountered by carers (data from Sanford, 1975)*

Problem	Frequency (per cent)	Percentage of carers able to tolerate problems
Sleep disturbance	62	16
Night wandering	24	24
Micturition	24	27
Incontinence of faeces	56	43
Incontinence of urine	54	81
Falls	58	52
Personality conflicts	26	54
Inability to wash and/or shave unaided	54	93

Speech disorders

Physiology

Cerebral dominance

The left hemisphere is said to be dominant for speech: 90 per cent of people are right-handed and have their speech centre in the left cerebral hemisphere. Of the 10 per cent who are left-handed, the majority still have their speech centre in the left hemisphere, but in the remainder the speech centre is in the right hemisphere (Rose and Capildileo, 1981). A major area controlling communication is the angular gyrus in the parietal lobe. This serves as an integration centre for all incoming sensory signals where visual, auditory, and tactile information is interpreted and related to language. (See Chapter 5, 'Rosemary'.)

Broca's area

Broca's area is in the frontal lobe near the motor cortex and is primarily responsible for the motor aspects of speech. This involves turning messages that are conceived in the brain into grammatically appropriate and smoothly coordinated speech patterns. Damage to Broca's area will cause the patient to have difficulty in finding words (*non-fluent dysphasia*).

Wernicke's area

Further back (posteriorly) in the temporal lobe is Wernicke's area where incoming communication is interpreted and messages are expressed in return. Damage to Wernicke's area causes a severe speech problem in that although his hearing is intact, the patient is unable to understand what is being said to him. With Broca's area intact, speech is fluent, but as the patient is unaware of his mistakes and grammatical errors, speech becomes unintelligible, and meaning, if any, is only conveyed in a roundabout way.

Knowledge of how different brain areas participate in the control of speech is not complete. The motor control of speech is governed from the area that controls speech muscles, but this is itself subject to control from other areas, mainly Broca's area; in turn this is intimately linked with parts of the parietal and temporal lobes, which are largely responsible for the intellectual aspects of speech (Ottoson, 1983).

Definitions

One of the factors creating a gulf between some of the health professionals who try to deal with the everyday problems of the person who has lost his use of language is the use of medical jargon. The several classifications of aphasia have hitherto all tended to fail to distinguish between the psychological, physiological and anatomical descriptions of speech and its disorders and to recognise the complexity of the relations between them. Traditionally, dysphasia was classified as *motor* (expressive) when there is difficulty in speaking due to a lesion in Broca's area – an anterior dysphasia. The terms 'sensory' or 'receptive' were used to describe difficulty in understanding resulting from a disorder of Wernicke's area, a posterior dysphasia. Fortunately, this classification has been superseded by the description of dysphasic disorders as non-fluent or fluent, which is much simpler as fewer terms are used.

Dysphasia

Dysphasia is a defect in the use of language, which may occur in comprehension, expression, reading or writing, although it usually affects all four. It is the result of damage to or dysfunction in the areas controlling speech in the dominant cerebral hemisphere.

Fluent dysphasia

A person with fluent dysphasia may have relatively normal speech but has difficulty in understanding what is being said to him. The individual with severe fluent dysphasia cannot appreciate or act on instructions and his attempts to speak are marred by uncorrected mistakes (*jargon dysphasia*). He fails both to understand and repeat the examiner's words but will suddenly start to chatter aimlessly and could be diagnosed as being confused or demented.

Non-fluent dysphasia

Here, an impairment in the production of speech can range from complete loss to shortened sentences and mild word-finding problems. Typically, the sentences are short, poorly formed and lack fluency. The patient has difficulty in the symbolic formulation of words, in expressing his thoughts by articulate sounds. He may be unable to find the appropriate word (*nominal aphasia*) or to enunciate polysyllabic words. In the more severe forms he is unable to make himself understood; his speech may be reduced to meaningless sounds or to an incomprehensible sequence of nominal and grammatical errors. The patient is frustrated and distressed by his disability. (See Chapter 5, 'Ronald'.)

It is uncommon for a patient to have a pure fluent or non-fluent dysphasia. More usually a mixed pattern is found, often with one type predominating. The type of dysphasia does not remain constant in an individual – during recovery, one type of dysphasia may evolve into another.

Global dysphasia

When both the production of speech and the comprehension of spoken and written language are impaired, this is described as *global dysphasia*. It often results from an extensive lesion of the dominant hemisphere involving both the frontal and temporal lobes.

The nurse who cannot communicate with her patient, particularly in a hospital situation when observed by other patients, is likely to feel an extreme sense of failure. Speech therapists can provide much needed advice and support.

Causes

The development of fluent speech depends upon normal hearing, normal intelligence and the ability to produce coordinated movements of the mouth, tongue and larynx. The nature of the speech disruption caused by neurological damage depends not only on the site and extent of the lesion, but also on when the insult occurs in the development of the individual.

The most common cause of dysphasia in later adult years is a vascular lesion, especially an ischaemic one. Transitory attacks of dysphasia may occur as a result of transient cerebral ischaemic episodes (TIAs). An intracranial tumour is the most common cause of dysphasia during the first half of adult life, and abscesses of the left temporal lobe and trauma of the speech areas of the brain also cause speech disorders. Non-fluent dysphasia results from a lesion in front of the lower end of the motor cortex, i.e. Broca's area. Fluent dysphasia may be caused by lesions scattered over a wide area of the temporoparietal lobes.

Dysarthria

Difficulty with articulation is known as *dysarthria*. A total inability to articulate is *anarthria*. The dysarthric patient is able to appreciate and formulate symbolic verbal constructions but he is unable to pronounce words in spoken language. Involuntary movement disorders that affect the tongue, lips or palate causing dysarthria are Parkinson's disease, chorea, Gilles de la Tourette's syndrome and tardive dyskinesia. (See Chapter 3, 'Movement disorders'.)

Multiple sclerosis

Many patients with multiple sclerosis experience some difficulty with speech. They may have difficulty in controlling the volume, quality and articulation of their speech, and irregularity and incoordination of phonation and respiration add to it. Dysarthria may be due either to spastic weakness or to ataxia of the muscles of articulation or to a combination of these factors. In the early stages articulation may be slurred; later, it may become explosive and almost unintelligible. 'Due to poor control of rhythm, there is a tendency to pronounce each syllable as if it is a separate word and to put the emphasis on the wrong syllables, some being pronounced too loudly and others too softly. In severe cases speech may become explosive and unintelligible, eventually with complete inability to articulate' (Espir and Rose, 1983).

Parkinson's disease

Speech disorders are present in many patients with Parkinson's disease. The main features are reduced intensity of voice, reduced variability of pitch, stress and rhythm (abnormality of prosody) and abnormal rates of speaking. The Parkinsonian patient may find that his voice becomes so soft (*dysphonia*) that the telephone cannot be used, thus causing problems at work, especially if the condition is accompanied by a mumbling repetition of certain syllables. A postal questionnaire of 261 members of the Parkinson's Disease Society revealed that only 94 (36 per cent) claimed to have 'no difficulty' with speech. Many patients and relatives referred to the distress and isolation caused by this handicap to communication (Gibberd et al, 1985).

Huntington's chorea

Chorea causes jerkiness of speech, sometimes with an explosive dysarthria due to sudden involuntary movements affecting the respiratory muscles of the larynx or mouth. When this is severe the patient's speech becomes unintelligible (Espir and Rose, 1983). Apart from difficulty in swallowing, progressive dysarthria in an intellectually normal patient may be very frustrating, particularly as a weakness of the hands may lead to an inability to write, cutting off all channels of communication. The patient often becomes distressed and frustrated when he is not understood. Lack of verbal communication, if allowed to develop, can cause the patient to become completely withdrawn from his environment. The longer the disease progresses the more speech symptoms patients may have, and speech, like performance in other areas, tends to fluctuate. One woman explained very clearly how she had been unhappy during a fortnight's admission to a Part III home because people could not understand her; she felt staff were too busy to listen to her efforts, and she had been embarrassed by an incontinence episode on account of this problem. Another man having great difficulty simply said to a nurse, 'Can't chat', although he was aware of the conversations occurring around him, and made friendly gestures.

Motor neurone disease

A patient may have severe dysarthria because of neuromuscular weakness, muscle wasting of tongue and cheeks, and weak lip closure. Lip and tongue sounds may be severely affected, with limited pitch and volume control causing difficulty in whistling. Excess salivation can interfere with sound projection and word formulation. Involvement of the larynx results in the voice becoming weak and monotonous. Speech becomes increasingly slurred. The soft palate may become immobile, causing speech to have a nasal sound due to nasal escape of air. The experienced nurse may need to explain to her junior colleague that the patient with motor neurone disease is clear in mind and thought, despite his increasing limitations of speech and movement.

Cerebrovascular accident

Loss and impairment of speech and language function are common features in patients who have had a cerebrovascular accident. A language difficulty due to the complexity of language function often persists long after the patient's physical recovery, although recovery is delayed if there is a communication barrier between the patient and the caring team. In the majority of patients the most obvious difficulty is finding words and using them articulately (non-fluent dysphasia). Their spoken language is full of hesitation and mispronunciation and any written language reflects the same problem. Comprehension of the written and spoken word is usually reasonably intact. About one-third of all patients who have had a cerebrovascular accident may have global dysphasia with gross comprehension difficulties and little spoken language. This occurs when there has been a massive mid-temporal lesion. Every patient produces a different combination and level of language difficulties and therefore different communication needs.

Wilson's disease

'A 12-year-old boy who had had hepatitis when he was 10 years old complained of stiffness across his shoulders; within 4 months, he could barely write or talk, and he exhibited flexion contractures of his right elbow and wrist' (Scheinberg and Sternlieb, 1984).

Speech in the Wilson's disease sufferer is generally difficult or impossible to understand, and requests for repetitions often frustrate the patient, who may angrily refuse to try to talk or may break into a long inspiratory gargling or a high-pitched cry. In an excellent book on Wilson's disease Scheinberg and Sternlieb (1984) explain that:

> Disturbances in speech trouble patients perhaps more than any other single neurological abnormality. In large part this is because the dysarthria is so frequently misinterpreted as a sign of mental retardation, which is ironic, since intelligence remains virtually unaffected in the great majority of patients. Either through disgust at having to repeat a phrase time after time before his listener understands, or because dystonic dysarthria makes intelligible speech virtually impossible, the patient may ultimately become completely mute.

Hearing loss

Anatomy and physiology

The human ear, like that of other mammals, has three distinguishable parts: the external, the middle, and the inner ear (Figure 2.1). The external ear consists of the portion

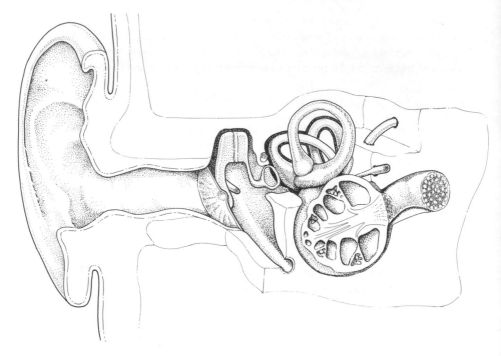

Figure 2.1   Audiovestibular mechanism (reproduced by kind permission of Duphar
Laboratories Ltd)

projecting from the side of the head, called the auricle or pinna, and the external
auditory canal, which ends blindly at the eardrum. The middle ear is a narrow, air-filled
space within the temporal bone, separated from the outside by the tympanic (eardrum)
membrane and crossed by a chain of three tiny bones: the auditory ossicles. The inner
ear is a complicated system of fluid-filled passages and cavities deep in the rock-hard
petrous portion of the temporal bone. It contains the sensory organs of hearing and
equilibrium, the specialised endings of the auditory or VIIIth cranial nerve.

Outer ear

The function of the outer ear is to collect sound waves and direct them inwards,
towards the middle and inner ear. Sound waves are conducted from the outer ear to the
oval window by vibrations of the drum, which are transmitted along the chain of
ossicles.

Middle ear

The middle ear is a small cavity in the temporal bone. When the tympanic membrane is
struck by sound waves it vibrates very rapidly, and the vibrations thus pass into the

middle ear. The Eustachian tube is a passage between the nasopharynx and the inner ear; it allows air to pass up from the nasopharynx into the middle ear on swallowing or yawning. The Eustachian tube has the function of keeping the external and internal air pressures equal. Provided that air can get up the Eustachian tube, there is air on both the inside and outside of the drum; this equal pressure enables the drum to vibrate freely. If the tube is blocked (as in nasal congestion) the pressure from inside the drum will be less than that on the outside and the drum will not be able to vibrate freely.

Stretched across the middle ear is a chain of tiny bones called the ossicles: the hammer (malleus), anvil (incus) and stirrup (stapes). They are joined together by moveable joints. When the eardrum vibrates the chain of ossicles is set in motion and allow sound waves to pass from the eardrum to the inner ear.

Inner ear

The inner ear has two parts: the cochlea, concerned with hearing, and the semicircular canals, concerned with the sense of balance. Vibrations in the outer chamber set up vibrations in the fluid of the middle chamber. Thus vibrations set up by sound waves outside the ear finally reach the cochlea and affect specially sensitive cells inside it. These cells form the organ of Corti. Surrounding the organ of Corti are endings of the nerve of hearing (acoustic nerve). The nerve fibres from the cochlea conduct impulses to the auditory nerve of the cerebral cortex.

Definitions

Deafness is loss of hearing, regardless of its severity. The effects depend on the severity of the loss, the rate of onset, whether one or both ears are affected and the age of onset. An adult who becomes very deaf does not lose his vocabulary but the lack of auditory feedback degrades his voice into a harsh flat monotone. Rapid total deafness in both ears is a catastrophe that affects every aspect of the victim's life, while gradually developing loss causes serious but less severe problems. In contrast, total loss of hearing in one ear is relatively trivial, regardless of age (Ludman, 1981).

Causes – acquired hearing loss

Conductive loss
   Obstructions – in the outer ear due to excessive wax or foreign bodies.
   Trauma – causing damage to the eardrum or the ossicles.
   Infections – from the nose and throat, e.g. colds, measles, tonsillitis.
   Otosclerosis – stapes immobilised by a growth of spongy bone.

Sensorineural loss
   Trauma – skull fracture or exposure to explosive blasts.
   Infections – mumps, chronic otitis media or meningitis.

Noise – prolonged exposure to noise (above 100 decibels).

Drugs – the antibiotics streptomycin and neomycin, or quinine.

Presbycusis – degeneration of hair cells and nerve fibres in the ear.

Menière's disease – a disorder of vestibular function of the inner ear.

Conductive loss

Conductive deafness arises from any impediment to the transmission of sound waves through the external canal and middle ear, as far as the footplate of the stapes.

The external auditory canal is most commonly obstructed by wax, but also by inflammation, e.g. a boil. Less commonly, congenital abnormalities and foreign bodies obstruct the canal.

The tympanic membrane (eardrum) may be ruptured by the penetration of a foreign body, by extension from a fracture of the skull base or by other events causing sudden compression. Pressure forces through the external auditory canal can occur in boxing, a hand slap, forceful syringing or a blow on the ear when the canal is filled with water as in water polo. Explosive blasts cause unilateral or bilateral perforation of the tympanic membrane accompanied by pain, tinnitus and vertigo.

Acute otitis media causes a severe throbbing headache, deafness and *tinnitus* (ringing in the ears). The patient, usually a child, will be pyrexial and the eardrum will show evidence of acute inflammation and may become perforated. Chronic otitis media causes deafness due to damage to the eardrum and middle ear.

The hair cells of the cochlea are normally able to respond to vibrations of the tympanic membrane. However, when the ossicular chain is immobilised by disease, as in otosclerosis, causing the stapes footplate to become fixed in the oval window, there is a hearing loss. This occurs in women more than men, from 15 to 30 years of age, often in a family with a history of deafness. Tinnitus may also be present.

Sensorineural loss

A sensory or perceptive loss refers to a defect somewhere in the cochlea. A neural loss results from a problem in the neural mechanism beyond the cochlea, e.g. the VIIIth nerve fibres. Because it can be difficult to identify precisely where the abnormality is, the term *sensorineural* is used to identify that the problem is somewhere beyond the oval window. The commonest cause of bilateral progressive sensorineural deafness is degeneration due to presbycusis, commonly occurring in elderly people.

Acute or chronic otitis media can develop from colds, measles, tonsillitis and other infections of the nose and throat. Some antibiotics, among them streptomycin and neomycin, irreversibly destroy cochlear hair cells. The hearing damage caused by large doses of salicylates is usually reversible. Some common diuretics, when given intravenously, may also be ototoxic.

Deafness may occur when a person has Menière's disease, which causes a rise of pressure in the inner ear, producing giddiness, nausea, vomiting and tinnitus. The deafness is often worse just before and after an attack, is gradually progressive and may be associated with gross distortion of normal sounds. When deafness is unilateral and progressive, it may be caused by an *acoustic neuroma*: a tumour of fibrous tissue that grows in the sheath of the acoustic nerve and compresses it, causing deafness, tinnitus and giddiness.

Involuntary movements

Distinctive types of spontaneous involuntary movements are a feature of many diseases of the nervous system. There are five main groups: tremor, chorea, myoclonus, tics and drug-induced dyskinesias. Abnormal involuntary movements are only physical signs and not diseases or pathological processes.

Tremor

Tremor is a rhythmical involuntary movement of part of the body. It may be classified either according to its frequency or whether it occurs at rest, on outstretching the hands or during movement. Postural, or action, tremor is most obvious when maintaining a position (e.g. holding the arms outstretched). Intention tremor occurs during active movement that is directed towards an object, e.g. in the finger–nose test or when trying to write.

Tremor is often the problem that brings the patient with Parkinson's disease to visit his or her doctor (i.e. it is the presenting sign). It becomes more marked when the patient is engaged in conversation or emotionally disturbed. The tremor may disappear on performing a voluntary movement and is absent during sleep. It usually begins in the fingers of one hand or arm, spreading to the foot of the same side and then to the opposite side and may appear only when the arm is held in a certain position. It only rarely occurs in the jaw or lips. At first the fingers flex and extend at the metacarpopharyngeal joints – when the thumb joins in, a pill-rolling movement results.

In the early stages of the disease, the tremor may only appear when the patient is tired or in stressful situations. At this stage, it is nothing more than a nuisance, causing embarrassment or awkwardness with fine movement and making certain tasks slow and laborious. As the disease progresses a stage is reached where the symptoms produce a definite disability, so that certain tasks have to be avoided altogether or can only be done at certain times of the day. (See Chapter 5, 'Frederick' and Frank'.)

Chorea

The first problem experienced by patients with either Huntington's chorea or Wilson's disease may be choreiform movements. Chorea consists of a series of unpredictable, forcible, rapid, irregular and unpatterned jerks, which are never integrated into a coordinated act: they are fleeting and usually exacerbated by voluntary movement and may present a rather comical, playful appearance. These movements may involve the fingers, the whole hand, or an entire extremity. They may be quick jerks, flinging motions or bizarre movements of one or more of the extremities. Not infrequently, muscles of the face are involved in choreiform movements, which therefore may include all types of grimacing or inappropriate smiling, pursing of the lips and sometimes protrusion of the tongue. Involuntary closure of the eyes (*blepharospasm*), rolling of the eyeballs, or a constant flinging about of the head may be included in these bizarre involuntary movements.

When the jerks are associated with complex voluntary movements the patient may appear 'fidgety' to the untrained observer. Gait and posture may be interrupted by abnormal movements. Walking is interrupted by lurches, stops and starts (the dancing gait); fine manipulations with hands, and speech and respiration, are similarly disturbed. Patients with chorea tend to cover up their disability by blending the pseudopurposeful choreic movements with normal voluntary movements.

Myoclonus

The term *myoclonus* is applied to a brief, shock-like muscular contraction, which may involve a whole muscle or may rarely be limited to a small number of muscle fibres. 'The muscle contraction is brief resembling an electric shock and cannot be controlled by will power' (Lees, 1985). Such myoclonic jerks are prominent in patients with sleep epilepsy, when they persist for up to an hour or so after waking. Myoclonus can also occur genetically, independent of epilepsy. Generalised myoclonic jerks are common following anoxic brain damage or with drug or alcohol withdrawal.

Tics

Tics are purposeless, stereotyped, and repetitive jerky movements, most commonly seen in the head and neck and, less commonly towards the periphery of the body. They mimic normal coordinated movements and may be temporarily suppressed by will power, often at the expense of mounting inner tension (Lees 1985).

The patients who have the most severe forms of tic may be sufferers of the Gilles de la Tourette syndrome, but there are also idiopathic and drug-induced tics and tics that occur in association with structural brain damage. Tics tend to be worse at times of anxiety, anger or self-consciousness. Some individuals find that their tics move to different muscle groups, while others have the same tic for years. Tics most often involve the face (blinking, sniffing, lip-smacking) and the upper arms (shoulder shrugging).

Drug-induced dyskinesia

A few years after the introduction of antipsychotic drugs into psychiatric practice in the early 1950s, reports began to appear of a persistent involuntary movement disorder associated with long-term administration: *tardive dyskinesia*. The disorder has been the subject of extensive debate and research for the last 30 years. Controversy continues to surround its diagnosis, incidence, underlying pathophysiology, relationship to antipsychotic drugs, prevention and treatment. The condition may affect both younger and older patients, regardless of sex. It has been diagnosed in people taking small doses for long and short periods, as well as in patients who take their medications irregularly. (See Chapter 5, 'Lesley'.)

Facial movements can include blinking of the eyes, lip-smacking, puckering, chewing and sucking mouth movements, as well as rolling, worm-like tongue movements with the mouth closed. There may be frequent head-nodding. Fingers and wrists may make sudden, non-rhythmic, purposeless, coarse, quick and jerky movements and the patient frequently crosses and uncrosses his legs, with slow twisting movements of the trunk (torsion movements). The grunting sounds that may occur are caused by involuntary movements of the diaphragm. These involuntary movements show considerable variation in severity, location and occurrence and they vary with the time of day and disappear with sleep. 'At the present time there is no known cure or consistently effective treatment for tardive dyskinesia' (Jewell and Chemij, 1983).

Rigidity and fatigue

Rigidity – Parkinson's disease

Patients with Parkinson's disease often complain of a feeling of stiffness: they may say, 'The rigidity is dull but constrained inertia, a tight and sluggish unresponsiveness to orders from the brain . . . It is like trying to swim in treacle – or rather, in jelly' (Godwin-Austen, 1984). The clinical examination provides evidence of rigidity of the muscles involved; those which should be soft and relaxed when not in use look 'rigid' because they are constantly tensed. This tightness and firmness can also be felt with the fingers when examining the patient. There is some resistance to passive motion around the elbow joint and sometimes in other joints – the wrist, knee, ankle and spine – and often a jerky quality to the resistance, as though the joint was moving through a series of gears: this is known as *cog-wheel rigidity*. Rigidity can predominantly affect the arm and leg on one side of the body or it may symmetrically involve all four limbs. The extent and severity of rigidity varies very considerably from one individual to another.

The rigidity cannot be eliminated at will, but under certain circumstances a rigid, hypokinetic patient may move very swiftly; for example, a patient with Parkinson's syndrome may move quickly to catch a ball suddenly thrown at him, and stories are told of bedridden rigid patients who jump up and run to safety to escape a fire. Periods of more or less severe muscular rigidity alternate with periods when the muscles are comparatively normal and relaxed; both phases vary in timing and duration (from minutes to hours) but changing from a rigid to a mobile state is usually abrupt (seconds). These states are totally involuntary: the patient cannot relax by an effort of will and in the rigid state it is extremely difficult to initiate a movement and equally hard to sustain motion once started.

Rigidity causes muscles to move slowly and during the early stages of the illness may give rise to aches, cramps and stiffness. Rigidity is often just as severe in the neck and trunk muscles compared with the limbs. The rigid patient tends to lose the righting reflexes that control posture and loss of balance will cause him to fall like a felled tree. In addition to frequent falls, rigidity may also cause difficulties with chewing, swallowing, coughing and all the activities of self-care.

The patient may be aware of the muscular rigidity not only as a sense of stiffness but as a tired, aching feeling, persistent soreness, a pain or a cramp. Rigidity of the spinal muscles causes back pain, which is aggravated by the tendency to stand leaning forward. Pain is usually associated with a general feeling of exhaustion and a disinclination to leave the favourite chair. Nevertheless, even when sitting still, the aching remains troublesome and is unrelieved by ordinary pain-killing tablets. This discomfort often gives rise to a distressing restlessness (Godwin-Austen, 1984).

Freezing – Parkinson's disease

Sudden episodes of immobility are a classical symptom of untreated Parkinson's disease, variously described as start-hesitation or freezing. In a study of 261 members of the Parkinson's Disease Society, 126 had 'freezing' (episodic severe immobility), 13 difficulty in starting walking and 115 difficulty in climbing stairs (Gibberd et al, 1985). The patient is abruptly riveted to the spot and cannot get moving again. While experienced most commonly during walking, such freezing episodes also affect speech, leading to sudden silence, during handwriting when the pen suddenly no longer crosses the page, and in many other manual motor acts such as playing a musical instrument, knitting or peeling potatoes.

In the case of long-standing Parkinsonism, of more than about 10 years' duration since onset, where rigidity and tremor have been very well controlled by medical therapy, freezing is often the cause of difficulty in daily activities. The greatest difficulty for such patients is to pass through narrow doorways. However, they may have no difficulty in walking up and down stairs steadily without hesitation or in stepping over an obstacle placed in front of them. Many patients may never have experienced freezing episodes before starting dopaminergic drugs, so their appearance for the first time during this treatment may be taken as an indication of the underlying pathology of the illness (despite drug therapy). It can also indicate that the treatment has to be altered in some way to bring about relief of the symptom.

Fatigue

Multiple sclerosis

Premature fatigue is one of the least understood symptoms of multiple sclerosis. Many sufferers are free of symptoms when at rest, but physical activities, such as running for a bus, or mowing the lawn, can bring on blurring of vision, unsteadiness, heaviness in the limbs and a sensation of extreme tiredness. This tiredness seems to have a quality of its own: during an attack of fatigue the sufferer is more obviously disabled, almost a different person. Fatigue is also produced or exacerbated by warm weather or hot baths.

Visual or sensory symptoms, and in particular multiple sclerosis fatigue, are hard for patients and close relatives to understand. It is important that doctors and nurses should give reassurance and an explanation so that everyone understands that the person with multiple sclerosis really is ill. The manual labourer will be unable to do his job without getting very tired exhausted. It may be more difficult to look after children who are young and active or impossible for a couple to enjoy an active sex life in quite the same way as before.

Myasthenia gravis

Myasthenia gravis is a disorder of neuromuscular transmission, characterised by muscle weakness and fatiguability. The major symptoms are weakness and fatiguability of skeletal muscles. The weakness may fluctuate considerably and is usually worse at the end of a day or after exercise. Any muscle group may be affected, but the initial symptoms are commonly confined to the extra-ocular muscles (eye closure and lid elevation). In addition, the muscles of facial expression, mastication, swallowing and speech are affected, as are the flexors and extensors of the neck and the muscles of the shoulder girdle. The patient's strength may be adequate to perform an initial movement, but on successive repetition, weakness becomes evident. During the medical examination, when the patient is asked to gaze upwards for a few minutes, his eyelids may droop down (ptosis), and holding his arms outstretched results in his arms drooping if the shoulder muscles are affected; and he is unable to count up to 20 or 30 as his voice fades away.

Parkinson's disease

Fatigue is the commonest of all symptoms in fully developed Parkinson's disease. Patients with Parkinson's disease have to make a very great effort to achieve what, to any normal person, would be ordinary physical exercise. The tiredness is not only a physical thing — it is mental as well. Lethargy and a disinclination to develop interests also form part of the disease. Sleep may restore vigour and many patients resort to an afternoon nap to provide strength for the end of the day. Another effect of fatigue is evident in the dramatic physical deterioration that may follow severe physical effort or great mental stress. It is as if such severe events exhaust the reserves of the patient, who then requires a period of rest to recover (Godwin-Austen, 1984).

Epilepsy

Some individuals are drowsy and sleep after a seizure. Emotional stress, fatigue, or major illnesses, particularly those associated with a high fever, are likely to increase seizure frequency. Drowsiness or sluggishness is a frequent side-effect of a new drug until the medication level is established. Also, excessive medication can produce drowsiness and physical as well as mental lethargy. Once the level is adjusted, these symptoms disappear.

Pain

The fatigue of pain is a result of many occurrences. Pain itself is fatiguing and there may be an underlying disease process that also physically depletes the patient. Some efforts to cope with pain, such as distraction, may further fatigue the patient. Muscle tension, which also adds to the fatigue, is a common, almost automatic response to pain. The degree of fatigue can sometimes be decreased considerably by utilising a relaxation technique regularly at intervals throughout the day.

Dizziness and vertigo

Patients' vocabulary

Many patients find it difficult to explain the many vague physical sensations associated with dizziness and will say that they experience a kind of giddiness, faintness, unsteadiness or light-headedness or a swaying feeling. Sensations of dizziness vary from a mild momentary episode with which the patient easily learns to live, to a violent and terrifying attack that leaves the person totally disabled. Extreme forms of dizziness are less vague in nature as they entail a subjective sensation of the patient moving or revolving in space or the illusion of objects moving past the patient. People say that they experience a feeling of an up and down of the body, of the floor coming up and of objects revolving round, everything spinning in circles, or a sudden falling feeling that throws them to the ground. Nausea, vomiting, pallor, sweating and *tachycardia* (rapid heart beat) are commonly observed in severe dizziness that starts suddenly.

Doctors' vocabulary

Gowers (1879) defined vertigo as 'any movement or sense of movement; whether in the individual himself or in external objects, that involves a defect, real or seeming, in the equilibrium of the body'. The Latin origin of the word 'vertigo' is 'vertere' meaning 'to turn', leading many doctors to use it to describe a rotary sensation. A patient is said to have vertigo when he or she feels that the surroundings are spinning round, either horizontally or vertically.

People who suffer from recurrent vertigo may have seen several doctors who have been unable to diagnose their complaint. This can result in great anxiety because they feel that no-one really understands their problem. There is, however, an elaborate array of diagnostic labels for a sudden onset of dizziness, combined with malaise, anxiety, apprehension, nausea and vomiting, that lasts for 2 or 3 days and where the sensation of vertigo is precipitated by sudden movements of the head: patients should therefore be advised to ask for a referral to a specialist. Even if the patient is offered a somewhat unpronounceable label such as 'episodic neurolabyrinthitis' or 'paroxysmal positional vertigo' or simply 'vestibular neuronitis', this is secondary to the fact that now he feels that somebody understands his problem; it has been identified and is therefore less frightening.

Mechanism of balance

All animals that walk on two legs, such as penguins, bears and humans, must control their centre of gravity all the time, for it changes with every step and every movement of the trunk and upper limbs. If we raise an arm in front of us, muscles of the trunk and both lower limbs must be brought into action to compensate for the change in the centre of gravity. If, for one reason or another, balance is suddenly lost and one begins to fall, a reflex action known as a 'righting mechanism' immediately comes into play in an attempt to regain equilibrium. This sense of loss of equilibrium, and the reflex mechanisms to regain and maintain it, are the function of the vestibular system. Many influences, scattered over the body, contribute to normal balance, and momentary disturbance of any one of them may cause minor giddiness. Balance is maintained by the interaction and coordination in the brain of nerve impulses from the inner ear, the eyes, the neck muscles and the limb joints.

The vestibular system lies in the brain stem and receives information from three main sources: the inner ear (semicircular canals, utricle and saccule), the eyes and the proprioceptive impulses. These all help to maintain a person's posture. The vestibule and semicircular canals are found in the inner ear and communicate with the cochlea. Movements of the head set up movements in the endolymph fluid of the canals and these act as stimuli to the nerve endings around the hair cells. These nerve endings serve as receptors and transmit the impulses to the brain.

The most important aspects of the anatomy and physiology of the vestibular system are the interrelationship of this system with the visual system, the proprioceptive sensory systems and multiple cerebral centres that are necessary for perfect balance, posture, locomotion, and eye movement control. From birth this information is integrated and stored in a data centre so that changes in body movement are tested against this learned pattern. Luxon (1984) points out that in unusual circumstances, e.g. skiing or sailing, these processes become conscious:

> The new information is 'foreign' to the data centre and may provoke unpleasant activity of the autonomic nervous system, such as nausea, vomiting, or sweating. This response continues until a new pattern of information is developed in the storage mechanism to 'recognise' the unusual input, and the process occurs continuously in daily life.

Vertigo

Vertigo is a hallucination of movement. Information concerning the position of the body reaches the central nervous system from a number of different pathways, including vision and a wide range of sensory receptors in the skin, joints and muscles. The vestibular system is concerned with detecting and transmitting acceleration; the semicircular canals are sensitive to angular acceleration while the otolith organ responds to linear acceleration, including gravitational forces. Vertigo is produced by diseases affecting the vestibular apparatus or its central connections. (See Chapter 5, 'Sheila'.)

The medical treatment of vertigo includes such contradictory measures as histamine stimulants, histamine blockers, vasoconstrictors, vasodilators and central nervous stimulants and depressants. In a review of 10 years' drug treatment of vertigo, Browning (1986) claimed that drugs were more commonly the cause of the problem than its solution: 'There appears from controlled studies to be no highly effective preparation for the vast majority of our patients and there is considerable individual variation in responsiveness and side-effects.' Vertigo caused by problems in the ear, neck or central pathways is usually made worse by head movement, so that patients tend to hold themselves very stiffly. Rehabilitation consists of a set of vestibular exercises, which can be learnt from physiotherapists.

Old age

Physiologically, there are contrasting views on what happens to the vestibular system with increasing age. It has been claimed that it remains unchanged, but some say that it is either enhanced or reduced with age. Whatever the cause of unfamiliar sensations of movement, their occurrence in elderly people is extremely frightening and unpleasant. A high proportion of elderly patients have degenerative cervical spondylosis, which could be made worse by osteoarthritis, chronic rheumatoid arthritis or osteoporosis. People who have poor vision, drop attacks or sensory neuropathy are particularly prone to falls, so it is not easy to know whether a person fell because of vertigo or through some other cause.

Head injury

Even though it may not start until a few days or weeks after the injury, the most common syndrome after head injury is vertigo whenever the person alters his position, particularly when lying down. Post-traumatic vertigo may result from a fracture of the temporal bone that affects the vestibular system.

Menière's disease

In 1860, Menière described this disease as a disorder characterised by recurrent attacks of vertigo associated with some hearing loss and tinnitus. It is a disorder of middle age, especially in the 50s. Usually, the person will have suffered from slowly progressive deafness and tinnitus in one or both ears for months or even years and then suddenly has an attack of giddiness. The giddiness may develop so rapidly that the patient may fall; more often, it takes a few minutes to become severe. In a severe attack the patient is literally prostrated and experiences an intense sensation of rotation of the surroundings. Vomiting soon develops, with severe nausea, and lasts for as long as the patient remains giddy. In the worst attacks the patient is helpless and presents an alarming case to onlookers.

In milder attacks prostration is less extreme and the patient may even be able to walk, although unsteadily. Deafness and tinnitus are sometimes intensified during the attack. The vertigo may last from half an hour to many hours and then gradually subside. On attempting to stand and walk the patient is unsteady and staggers. In the intervals between attacks giddiness is occasionally brought on by sudden movements of the head. The attacks tend to recur at irregular intervals, although they may be aggravated by stress or emotional upset, and occur in bouts interspersed with spontaneous remissions, which may last for as long as 4 years. The patient must rest during an attack, lying perfectly still. There is no one treatment that will satisfy all patients. The four main symptoms – vertigo, distortion of hearing, tinnitus and the psychological aspects of the condition – have to be given an equal share of attention. It is not always the same symptom that chiefly occupies the patient's attention but nurses and doctors have to know which problem is his main concern. Most often it is vertigo, but this in itself causes psychological effects. In a few, it is the deafness or associated distorted hearing that is the main worry, particularly in those whose occupation involves public speaking or performing as a musician. Patients may be advised to restrict their salt intake, they may be given diuretics and vitamin supplements, and the doctor may utilise medication that aims to improve inner ear circulation and control fluid pressure changes of the inner ear chambers.

Pain

Psychology

The patient who has frequent attacks of pain may become so involved in trying to minimise or prevent them that he has little time or energy left to enjoy his life or form adequate and fulfilling relationships; he neglects his family and, ultimately, himself. As the migraine sufferer's body tends to react quickly and in an exaggerated fashion to actual or potential stress, relaxation therapy can help some people. Psychological disturbances do not themselves cause migraine. Anxiety and depression often aggravate migraine and may also add to the burden, causing tension headaches. Most patients with tension headaches are aware that they never completely relax and it is this inability to relax the muscles of the face, scalp and neck that is one of the main features of their condition. The pain in tension headache is made worse by drugs that constrict the blood vessels and is temporarily relieved by substances such as alcohol that dilate the vessels (Wilkinson, 1976).

Factors affecting pain (Budd, 1982)

- The original lesion that produces the pain.
- Personality of the patient – anxiety, depression, hysteria, obsessional traits or a tendency to hypochondriasis all make pain worse.
- Personal concept of the problem.
- Response to current and past therapy.
- Rapport with the therapeutic team.
- Attitudes of other people to the illness – whether they are sceptical or supportive.
- Prognosis, whether known or unknown.
- Personal pressures – social, economic and family.

Cultural influences

People from widely divergent backgrounds tend to use the same words to describe their pain. Some cultural groups expect an extravagant display of emotion in the presence of pain; others value stoicism, restraint and the playing down of their symptoms. Zborowski (1952) found that northern and western European races exhibit less emotion and complain less when in pain than southern European or Latin races. Both Italians and Jews tended to be very emotional in response to pain and to exaggerate their pain experience, leading some doctors to conclude that they had a lower threshold of pain than other groups. An Irish person may prefer to ignore and deny or play down the presence of pain because of an 'oppressive sense of guilt', which is said to be a feature of Irish culture. The Italians could be dismissed as 'overemotional' by the nurse who values stoicism and restraint and the Irish might have their suffering ignored as they continually underplay it. The factor governing behaviour for all groups seems to be the level of approval given for the public expression of pain and emotion (Melzack and Torgerson, 1971).

Zborowski (1952) also found different attitudes towards the pain process itself in people from various cultural backgrounds. Italians were mainly concerned with the immediacy of the pain sensation. When in pain they complained a great deal, drawing attention to their suffering by groaning, moaning or crying. However, once they were given analgesics and the pain wore off, they forgot their suffering and returned to normal behaviour. By contrast, Jewish patients were mainly concerned with the meaning and significance of the pain 'in relation to their health, welfare and, eventually, for the welfare of their families'. Their anxieties were concentrated on the implications for the future of the pain experience, focusing on the cause of the pain rather than relieving the actual pain itself.

Observing the patient

Patients with chronic pain do *not* usually display intensive muscle and autonomic nervous system responses. However, when these are present the nurse should observe and record what she sees.

Skeletal muscle responses to pain (Bourbonnais, 1981):

1. *Body movements*: immobility; purposeless or inaccurate body movements; protec-tive movements, including withdrawal reflex, rhythmic or rubbing movements.
2. *Facial expression*: clenched teeth, wrinkled forehead, biting of lower lip, widely opened or tightly shut eyes.

The autonomic nervous system also responds to the presence of pain with visible signs:

3. *Sympathetic nervous system activation*: increased pulse, respiration, diastolic and systolic blood pressure; cold perspiration; pallor; dilated pupils; nausea; muscle tension.
4. *Parasympathetic activation in some visceral pain*: Low blood pressure; slow pulse.

Migraine

The word 'migraine' comes from the Greek term for a one-sided headache. Not all headaches are due to migraine and since the treatment will depend on the cause, it is important to separate the different types of headache. Headache can be due to conditions within the skull, outside the skull or general disease of the body or mind. The medical significance of headache varies widely as the causes themselves range from relatively minor emotional difficulties to serious illness.

Classical migraine

Some people experience a warning of the impending headache consisting of disturbance of vision with flashing lights or an inability to see a certain area of the visual field for 20–30 minutes. There may be a feeling of unusual well-being that develops gradually or over a 10–30-minute period: it clears more rapidly than it develops and shortly afterwards the headache begins. Others experience symptoms of drowsiness, hunger and constipation or slight looseness of the bowels on the day of the migraine attacks. The headache can last for minutes or for more than a day and be accompanied by abdominal and/or visual symptoms, but while the headache is present, the patient has a dislike of bright light and many experience difficulty in focusing. In a severe attack sufferers often lose their appetite, suffer nausea and vomit.

Common migraine

This term describes a bilateral headache located behind the eyes, in the temples or at the back of the head. It is usually not preceded by an aura; nausea and vomiting may occur if the headache is severe, but less often and less severely than in classical migraine. The common migraine patient may have daily headaches for years, while the classical migraine sufferer is frequently pain-free between his attacks.

Tension headache

This is a common type of headache and is produced by anxiety, depression, aggression and frustration. It occurs in the frontal, temporal, parietal and occipital regions and in the neck and can be unilateral or bilateral. The headache may be a dull ache or a feeling of constriction or pressure. It is attributed to long-sustained contraction of the frontalis and occipital muscles in the scalp or of muscles in the face and neck. (See Chapter 5, 'Ann' and 'Betty'.)

Headache stigma

Many sufferers are reluctant to admit they have migraine. They are convinced that others will not believe them or that doctors will tell them that it is all in their minds or that they are 'neurotic' (Evans, 1978).

Headache

Myths

Because migraine is so little understood, it is not surprising that myths have grown up about the incidence of the condition and the characteristics of the sufferers. A great deal of nonsense has been written about a 'migraine personality', including details about attitudes, ambitions and frustrations of migraine sufferers. It was once considered a mark of intellect and sensitivity to be a migraine sufferer. However, research shows that migraine may affect people of any class, age, occupation, creed or race, although those who seek specialist help may tend to be more of middle-class than of lower socio-economic groups.

> *Sinus*:   sinus conditions rarely if ever produce headaches.
> *Vision*:   headaches are rarely caused by visual acuity or muscular imbalance.
> *High blood pressure*:   most patients with hypertension do not have headaches.
> *Constipation*:   does not cause headache.
> *Intellectuals*:   legend has suggested that the migraine sufferer is more intelligent
>   than average, but studies dispute this (Freese, 1976).
> *Allergies*: in practice, it is not easy to establish that a particular food causes a
>   headache in a susceptible individual (Critchley, 1980).

Facts

A headache is not a disease: it is a complaint, a symptom. Not everyone's attack is identical and some may be quite bizarre. Headaches are often caused by psychological factors after a head injury.

Trigger factors

These are many and various. They may be dietary, endocrine, psychological, physical or associated with changes in the environment, including:

- gardening, or any unusual bending or stooping;
- any unusual physical or mental activity, however much enjoyed;
- lifting heavy weights or straining;
- late rising at weekends or on holiday;
- change of routine;
- climatic change;
- high winds;
- noise;
- certain foods, e.g. alcohol and cocoa derivatives;
- bright light;
- travel;
- certain smells;
- shock;
- emotion;
- overfatigue.

Cluster headache

Cluster headaches are a distinctive syndrome in which the pain is one-sided, and may affect either eye and the adjacent area of the head. Attacks are more common in men than in women and they start later in life, usually in the third, fourth or fifth decades. They occur far more regularly than migraines, coming in clusters and lasting for about 30–60 minutes. The pain characteristically develops during sleep and may last for several hours, recurring at the same time each day. The headaches recur in one or more daily bouts in clusters for a period of weeks or months, separated by long intervals of complete freedom. The pain remains localised behind one eye, which goes red, and there is often congestion of the nostril on that side (Evans, 1978). (See Chapter 5, 'Bob'.)

The neuralgias

There are several pain syndromes associated with peripheral nerve damage that are generally known as neuralgic pain. They are characterised by severe, unremitting pain, which is difficult to alleviate. The causes of neuralgic pain include viral infections of nerves, nerve degeneration associated with diabetes, poor circulation in the limbs, vitamin deficiency and ingestion of poisonous substances such as arsenic. Almost any infection or disease that produces damage to peripheral nerves, particularly the large myelinated nerve fibres, may be the cause of pain that is labelled as neuralgic. (See Chapter 5, 'Carl'.)

Trigeminal neuralgia

Neuralgia is paroxysmal pain radiating in the area supplied by a sensory nerve and it frequently affects the trigeminal nerve to produce the condition of trigeminal neuralgia. The trigeminal (Vth cranial nerve) provides sensory fibres to the face and scalp and motor fibres to the muscles of the jaw. Trigeminal neuralgia may occur as a symptom of underlying neurological disease such as multiple sclerosis or meningioma or other cerebral tumours. Severe trigeminal neuralgia may lead to weight loss and general debility.

In an attack, the patient suddenly freezes with an intensely painful expression, usually making no sound. He stops everything he is doing while he concentrates on his pain, then straightens up and continues the conversation. The attacks of burning stabbing pains in the face travel along the course of one or more branches of the nerve. The pain is extraordinarily intense but brief and may occur frequently. It may be triggered off by a touch or a trigger point on the face, eating, washing, a cold wind or by movements of the facial muscles. The simple act of talking triggered pain in one patient to such an extent that he had to resort to written answers. Gentle stimulation can trigger pain, whereas severe pinches, pin jabs or intense pressure fail to evoke it. The syndrome commonly has its onset in middle or later life, in people living in cold countries, and most often affects the right side of the face. (See Chapter 5, 'Doreen'.)

Post-herpetic neuralgia

Infection by the *Varicella zoster* virus causes both chickenpox, usually in children, and inflammation of one or more sensory nerves, usually in patients over 50 years. The inflammation, which is painful, is associated with eruptions (*shingles*) on the skin at the termination of the nerve. The herpetic attack is itself painful but the pain usually subsides. In a small number of people, however, the post-herpetic pain persists and may become worse. The neuralgic skin area is extremely hyperaesthetic so that the pain is aggravated by any stimuli applied to the skin: even the friction of clothes is highly unpleasant and contact is avoided as much as possible. The pain may also be intensified by noise in the immediate vicinity or by emotional stress.

This condition may last for many months or even years and is very difficult to treat.

Carpal tunnel syndrome

This syndrome, one of the most common disorders affecting the peripheral nerves, results from long-standing compression of the median nerve as it passes the transverse carpal ligament. This process is more common in women than in men and produces symptoms of pain, burning, numbness and tingling. The pain is more severe after the hands have been used for activities such as knitting, peeling vegetables or wringing clothes. The pain is almost always worse at night and probably results from unconscious flexion while asleep. The patient will notice that she is unable to move the thumbs through the full range of motion because the thumb muscles have atrophied. (See Chapter 5, 'Elizabeth'.)

Dysphagia

Dysphagia is the subjective sensation of food sticking in the throat when swallowing. Swallowing is activated by the stimulus of food or by stimulation of the areas supplied by the trigeminal nerve; it is an act that begins voluntarily but ends as a reflex. Swallowing is a complicated reflex action, the initial stages of which are under voluntary control, so that it is absent in the unconscious patient. Masticated or chewed food, as well as a collection of saliva, is called a bolus. The reflex is initiated by compressing the bolus between the tongue and the hard palate, thus pushing solids into the pharynx and squirting them and liquid down into the lower oesophagus.

Difficulty with these first two stages of swallowing is caused by neuromuscular disorders such as motor neurone disease, multiple sclerosis, paralysis of the lower bulbar nerves and infection of the bulbar neurones in acute poliomyelitis. Dysphagia is commonly seen for a few days after a stroke.

As a symptom, it may merely cause embarrassment and disruption of the person's social life and the fear of eating in public, but it may threaten existence by causing starvation or respiratory complications. When a patient has difficulty in swallowing, this limits the provision of well-balanced nourishing food, which may need to be liquidised and yet relate to the person's dietary preferences.

Parkinson's disease

Patients with Parkinson's disease have motility problems, both in the pharynx and the oesophagus. Saliva pools in the mouth and drooling is common. Swallowing disorders have been reported several times, one study finding these in 50 per cent of Parkinson patients. The characteristic features of the Parkinsonian swallow include tongue tremor, hesitancy in initiating swallowing, difficulty in bolus formation and disturbances of pharyngeal motility. Parkinson patients may be silent aspirators with decreased cough reflexes and lack of awareness of aspiration. Although six patients in one study demonstrated disordered swallowing, only three of them admitted to having any difficulty in swallowing (Croker et al, 1982).

Myasthenia gravis

The muscles supplied by the cranial nerves are usually those first affected. Therefore, difficulty with chewing, swallowing and holding up the head, as well as nasal regurgitation, may occur early in the disease. The palatal, pharyngeal and upper oesophageal muscles are eventually involved in 40 per cent of all patients with myasthenia. The degree of involvement varies between patients and in individual patients. In some cases milder symptoms are ignored so that the patient first visits his doctor with severe pharyngeal involvement that results in difficulties with handling secretions. Weakness of masseter and temporal muscles and orofacial weakness result in difficulty with chewing and enunciating.

Motor neurone disease

Here, weakness of the facial muscles may be accompanied by weakness of the muscles of mastication supplied by the trigeminal nerve. In these circumstances the patient has difficulty in chewing food and in keeping it from collecting between teeth and cheeks. Atrophy of the tongue muscles makes it difficult to move the food into the pharynx to initiate swallowing. In some cases rapidly progressive weight loss is associated with accelerating weakness (Norris et al, 1985). In one study of problems in 42 patients with motor neurone disease, slurring occurred in 28 (67 per cent), choking in 24 (57 per cent) and drooling in 21 patients (50 per cent) (Newrick and Langton-Hewer, 1984).

Huntington's chorea

In some patients with Huntington's chorea the swallowing mechanism is affected, whereas with others salivation is a problem. When this occurs the patient needs frequent reminders to swallow and thus clear his mouth; medication may ease drooling problems. Eating and gaining enough nourishment are problems that become increasingly difficult as the disease progresses, so that in the later stages people are invariably emaciated. Drooling and messy eating may be the main problem area and the patient may choose to eat apart from his family because they are upset by the mess.

Stroke

Difficulties with feeding and swallowing and a fear of choking may cause more distress and anxiety during the early recovery stages after a stroke than the loss of other functions. The normal guarding mechanism in the airway prevents the inhalation of solids or liquids into the lungs and is essential for survival. The neuromuscular mechanism that normally warns us that something is about to be swallowed may be lost and the various muscle groups involved may fail to function so that foreign matter enters the lungs directly. The muscle groups may fail to pass on the bolus of food completely so that during the next inspiration the debris is carried into the lungs. Breath control may be lost and simultaneous inspiration and swallowing in the adult is very dangerous.

The loss of facial nerve function of the lips and cheeks on the affected side will cause the angle of the mouth to drop. A patient may be unaware that his lips are not closed and swallowing is very difficult with the lips and teeth separated, especially if the tongue is also weak. Loss of the function of the cheeks allows food debris to accumulate.

The patient who has had a cerebrovascular accident may be unable to appreciate the presence of saliva, bland fluids, water at body temperature or semisolids with sufficient accuracy to move the bolus around the mouth to prepare it for swallowing. Loose dentures get dislodged and a lower denture could become lodged in the pharynx. The patient may be unaware when his lower jaw has dropped away from the upper and therefore cannot swallow under these conditions.

Although the first part of the swallowing mechanism is normally under voluntary control, it has become semiautomatic in the healthy adult and requires little conscious effort. For the patient who has had a cerebrovascular accident, this complex action is no longer so easy and he will need specific rehabilitation efforts directed towards regaining this action of his soft palate and pharynx as a safe and comfortable process.

Facial paralysis

The VIIth cranial nerve, the facial nerve, is that most commonly affected by disease. A complete facial paralysis causes considerable difficulty with eating and drinking. During meals food tends to collect between teeth or dentures and the cheek and spill out of the side of the mouth.

Practical tips – feeding

Judicious use of liquidised food and the avoidance of strong spices and irritating food and drink are helpful to the person with impaired swallowing and aspiration. When a nurse or carer at home assists with feeding the patient should be seated upright with his feet flat on the floor either on a dining-type chair, or in a wheelchair and brought as near as possible to the table. When being fed, a small table with the helper seated opposite is ideal. It is important that whoever feeds the dysphagic person has a calm manner and allows plenty of time for the task. Many mute patients will obey verbal instructions. While feeding very small amounts of food at a time, encouragement can be given to the patient to chew a bit more, close his mouth, hold his breath and try to swallow when he feels ready. The patient who chokes can be dealt with by using the abdominal thrust, or Heimlich manoeuvre, to compress the lungs until the resultant pressure forces the obstruction from the airway, by giving the patient a quick hug from behind, pressing the fists into his abdomen with an upward thrust.

Wilson's disease

Within months after a bout of jaundice at age 19, a 'wild expression,' flexion contactures of the hands, drooling, open-mouthedness, dysphagia and mutism developed in a woman. The handwriting of a 15-year-old girl, which had been notably beautiful, deteriorated suddenly. Soon thereafter an awkward stance, a jaw that hung open, and difficulty in swallowing liquids developed (Scheinberg and Sternlieb, 1984).

The patient with Wilson's disease finds that when speech problems begin to get worse, he has difficulty in swallowing. Eventually the immobility of his tongue is such that food placed in his mouth cannot be manipulated and delivered to the oropharynx. Scheinberg and Sternlieb (1984) explain that 'Interference with swallowing — caused in part by the hypertonia and spasm of mouth, throat and neck musculature — may be so severe that tube feeding is necessary'.

Problems with sexuality

Disability

In our ageist culture we have negative views of sexuality in the elderly and the sexual problems of the physically disabled are only beginning to be recognised and discussed.

Studies of the chronically ill or disabled have shown that sexual activity is particularly susceptible to change. Whenever illness causes a reduction in physical sensitivity and even when a good physical recovery occurs, a large proportion of patients reduce their sexual activity. Sexual functioning and drive may not be impaired but the indirect effects of disability may make intercourse difficult or impossible. These effects include pain, the partner's fear of inflicting pain, fear of the medical consequences of intercourse and either uncontrollable body movements or paralysis. Some people automatically expect others to withdraw from physical, emotional and social contact because of the new body that they now inhabit, which is 'scarred' by some form of disability; there is a fear of rejection. One patient explained that: 'It is extraordinarily difficult to make love satisfactorily if both lovers are in wheelchairs'. Some drugs prescribed for particular impairments have side-effects that reduce libido or potency.

Although it is generally accepted that sexual difficulties are a common accompaniment of neurological disability, their exact frequency is not well known. In patients with spinal cord injury sexual function is almost invariably affected initially. However, to what degree this occurs is dependent on the nature of the cord lesion. Some return of function is likely within a year of the injury. Miller et al (1965) found that in a series of 297 people with multiple sclerosis, 62 per cent of the men were impotent. Two-thirds of these, all of whom had urinary symptoms, were thought to have a physical cause for their impotence. In this study, women were less prepared to answer the questions about sexual intercourse than were the men.

In the long term problems of sexuality may still be a serious worry to patients or their relatives and this may either be because of increased or decreased sexuality, or because of a personality change when the partner who has been unaffected may feel physically or mentally repelled. In such circumstances, specialist advice should be sought where possible and organisations exist to provide this help. Nurses should attempt not to appear shocked by the questions and actions of patients but try to correct them reasonably. However, if they feel that it is beyond their competence to deal with, they should ensure that the message is passed on and the problems are not suppressed, later to emerge as bigger ones.

For many patients sexual performance is perhaps not as important as the feeling of being loved, accepted and respected. Counselling and advice on sexual problems should involve the sexuality of the whole person as well as aspects of genital sex. Relatives may find it helpful to discuss these problems with others at self-help groups. The nurse's role in helping patients in the area of sexuality is to be able to identify problems and intervene appropriately by teaching or counselling within the limits of her knowledge, or by referring patients or clients to specialist practitioners or agencies for help.

Cerebrovascular accident

Many studies report difficulties of sexual function following stroke and in a proportion of cases complete cessation of sexual activities occurs (Newman, 1984). In a study of 67 stroke patients living at home with a regular partner and sexually active until the day of the stroke, about one third maintained their frequency of intercourse, one third reduced their frequency and the remaining one-third ceased sexual relations. The cessation of sex was influenced by loss of sensation on the affected side (Fugl-Meyer and Jaaski, 1980).

The patient's personality may have changed as a result of the stroke. The nurse may hear spouses say, 'He's not the man I married.' How can they be expected to be intimate with someone who is, in effect, a stranger? The spouse may now find the physical appearance of the partner repulsive. Sexual enjoyment may be reduced because of motor or sensory impairment. If the patient is very dependent on his spouse, much of the magic may go out of the relationship: 'I have to wash him, bath him, powder him and wipe his bottom: how can I look upon him as a lover?' Sexual problems may be a reflection of a general breakdown of marriage that may occur after any disabling illness (Mulley, 1985).

Head injury

Often one of the greatest problems for both male and female brain-damaged patients, especially those in the younger age group, is that of disinhibition. It is sometimes more obvious in male patients, who can then be especially difficult in mixed company. The altered behaviour may range from the very mild backchat frequently experienced by nursing staff who care for patients in orthopaedic wards, to the more unacceptable and determined attempts by patients to force the nursing staff to have some form of sexual intercourse, or it may take the form of sexual encounters between patients, either of the same or the opposite sex.

Multiple sclerosis

Multiple sclerosis is a disease of young adults. Changing sexual response is of frequent concern to men who become impotent and to women who lose sensation in the perineal region.

A person who has very severe functional impairment needs almost total physical care, and the physical dependency produced leads to a complete restructuring of social roles and undermines the sense of reciprocal value in a marital relationship. Robinson (1988) describes one marriage where 'She has lost control of her body and her sexuality, and he has become a constant and intimate body "maintenance man". In the process both of them appear to be struggling – not very successfully – to sustain their essential selves independently to the crumbling physical shell of her body'.

Incontinence is still a topic shrouded in embarrassing silence. Simply by being incontinent, having to wear special pants and pads or being catheterised, a person must feel less attractive.

'The way we see and judge ourselves and others as attractive, worthwhile, independent and social beings in our working, caring and leisure activities are all dimensions of sexuality' (Webb, 1984). Incontinence is, as Robinson says, 'Associated with the asexual world of the very young or the very old', so that 'Special efforts must be made to sustain a clear identity with its onset. Although this symptom may be concealed or negotiated around in public – perhaps with difficulty – it cannot readily be hidden in intimate personal relationships.'

A study took place in four London boroughs to determine how many patients with urinary symptoms due to neuropathic bladder experienced difficulties with sexual intercourse (Glover and Thomas, 1986). Such difficulties were reported by 65 of the 136 patients with multiple sclerosis and by 31 of the 49 patients with other neurological diseases. Difficulties were reported more commonly by men than by women. The problems were sufficient to prevent intercourse in 61 of the 96 cases reporting difficulties, although only four said that it was their bladder symptoms alone that prevented them having intercourse.

Webb (1985) says that 'Nurses who are skilled communicators offer an important supportive service in a warm and non-judgemental manner to patients needing to talk about their feelings and problems.' Some couples need factual information only, mainly of a physical or a practical nature, which they are then usually able to put into effect. Others need advice as to which of several possible solutions to their problem is likely to be the most appropriate for them. 'Husbands are frequently concerned about intercourse after the wife has an indwelling catheter drainage. There is no reason to discourage sexual intercourse simply because the women is catheterized' (Wolf, 1980). Nurses in all specialities, in both institutional and community care, should recognise patients' sexual as well as other human needs. Occasionally, the situation becomes so difficult that they need sexual counselling by an expert, which can be arranged through the organisation Sexual Problems of the Disabled (SPOD). (See Chapter 4, 'Chronic illness'.)

References

Bourbonnais F (1981) Pain assessment: development of a tool for the nurse and the patient. *Journal of Advanced Nursing*, 6(4): 277–282.

Browning G G (1986) Medical treatment of vertigo. In: *Current Approaches: Vertigo*, Downey L J (ed.), pp. 48–52. Eastbourne: Duphar Laboratories.

Budd K (1982) *Pain*. London: Update Publications.

Critchley E (1980) *Pocket Guide to Migraine and Headaches*. London: Arlington.

Croker J R (1982) Dysphagia. *Geriatric Medicine*, 12(2): 71–2, 75–6.

Espir M L E and Rose C F (1983) *The Basic Neurology of Speech*, 3rd edn. Oxford: Blackwell Scientific.

Evans P (1978) *Mastering your Migraine*. London: Granada.

Freese A S (1976) *Headaches: The Kinds and Cures*. London: Allen and Unwin.

Fugl-Meyer A and Jaasko L (1980) Post-stroke hemiplegia and sexual intercourse. *Scandinavian Journal of Rehabilitation and Medicine*, Supplement 7: 158–166.

Gibberd F B, Oxtoby M and Jewell P F (1985) The treatment of Parkinson's disease – a consumer view. *Health Trends*, 17(1): 19–21.

Glover D and Thomas T (1986) Urinary symptoms and sexual difficulties. *Nursing Times*, 82(14): 72–75.

Godwin-Austen R (1984) *The Parkinson's Disease Handbook*. London: Sheldon Press.

Gowers W R (1879) *Manual of Diseases of the Nervous System*, 2nd edn. London: J A Churchill.

Harding A E (1985) Degenerative disorders. In: *Neurology*, Ross Russell R W and Wiles C M (eds.), pp. 187–203. London: Heinemann Medical.

Jewell J A and Chemij M (1983) Tardive dyskinesia, the involuntary movement disorder that no one really understands. *Canadian Nurse*, 79(6): 20–24.

Lees A J (1985) *Tics and Related Disorders*. Edinburgh: Churchill Livingstone.

Ludman D (1981) ABC of neurology: difficulty in swallowing. *British Medical Journal*, 282(1): 799–801.

Luxon L M (1984) The anatomy and physiology of the vestibular system. In: *Vertigo*, Dix M R & Hood J D (eds.), pp. 1–36. Chichester: John Wiley and Sons.

Melzack R and Torgerson W S (1971) On the language of pain. *Anesthesiology*, 34: 50–59.

Miller H, Simpson C A and Yeates W K (1965) Bladder dysfunction in multiple sclerosis. *British Medical Journal*, 1: 1265–1269.

Mulley G P (1985) *Practical Management of Stroke*. Beckenham: Croom Helm.

Newman S (1984) The social and emotional consequences of head injury and stroke. *International Review of Applied Psychology*, 33: 427–455.

Newrick P G and Langton-Hewer R (1984) Motor neurone disease; can we do better? A study of 42 patients. *British Medical Journal*, 289(2): 539–542.

Norris F H, Smith R A and Denys E H (1985) Motor neurone disease: towards better care. *British Medical Journal*, 291(2): 259–262.

Ottoson D (1983) *Physiology of the Nervous System*. London: Macmillan.

Pinching A J (1986) Clinical and immunological aspects of AIDS. Unpublished Sandoz Lecture. London: National Hospital for Nervous Diseases.

Robinson I (1988) *Multiple Sclerosis*. London: Routledge and Kegan Paul.

Rose F C and Capildeo R (1981) *Stroke: The Facts*. Oxford: Oxford University Press.

Sanford J R A (1975) Tolerance of debility in elderly dependents by supporters at home: its significance for hospital practice. *British Medical Journal*, 3: 471–473.

Scheinberg I H and Sternlieb I (1984) *Wilson's Disease*. Philadelphia: W B Saunders.

Walton J N (1977) *Brain's Diseases of the Nervous System*, 8th edn., p. 1181. Oxford: Oxford University Press.

Webb C (1984) How would you feel? *Nursing Times*, 80(6), *Community Outlook*: 45–46.

Webb (1985) *Sexuality, Nursing and Health*. Chichester: John Wiley and Sons.

Wilkinson M (1976) *Living With Migraine*. London: Heinemann Medical.

Wolf J K (1980) *Practical Clinical Neurology*. New York: Henry Kimpton.

Zborowski M (1952) Cultural components in response to pain. *Journal of Social Issues*, 8: 16–30.

Further reading

Dementia

World Health Organisation (1986) *Dementia in Later Life: Research and Action.* Geneva: World Health Organisation.

Adams T (1987) Dementia is a family affair. *Nursing Times,* **83**(5): *Community Outlook,* 7–9.

Corker E (1982) Strained relations. *Nursing Mirror,* **155**(4): 32–34.

McArthur J H and McArthur J C (1986) Neurological manifestations of autoimmune deficiency syndrome. *Journal of Neuroscience Nursing,* **18**(5): 242–249.

Moir-Bussy B (1983) Creutzfeld–Jakob disease. *Nursing Times Journal of Infection Control Nursing Supplement,* Supplement 19, 16–19.

Speech

Bedford J (1985) Bridging the communication gap. *Nursing Times,* **81**(5), 22–23.

Brian R (1965) *Speech Disorders: Aphasia, Apraxia and Agnosia,* 2nd edn. London: Butterworth.

Perry A R, Gawel M and Rose F C (1981) Communication aids in patients with motor neurone disease. *British Medical Journal,* **282**(1): 1690–1692.

Scott S and Caird F I (1984) The response of the apparent receptive speech disorder of Parkinson's disease to speech therapy. *Journal of Neurology, Neurosurgery and Psychiatry,* **47**(3): 302–304.

Scott S, Caird F I and Williams B O (1985) *Communication in Parkinson's Disease.* Beckenham: Croom Helm.

Thrush J (1981) Communicating with patients with speech problems. *British Medical Journal,* **282**(1): 802–803.

Hearing loss

Ballantyne J and Martin J A M (1984) *Deafness,* 4th edn. Edinburgh: Churchill Livingstone.

Lysons K (1984) *Hearing Impairment: A Guide for People With Auditory Handicaps and Those Concerned With Their Care and Rehabilitation.* Cambridge: Woodhead-Faulkner.

Youngson R (1986) *How To Cope With Tinnitus and Hearing Loss.* London: Sheldon Press.

Involuntary movements

Hudgson P (1983) Writer's cramp. *British Medical Journal,* **286**(1): 585–586.

Dizziness and vertigo

Ludman H (1981) Vertigo. *British Medical Journal,* **282**(1): 454–457.

Luxon L M (1984) Vertigo in old age. In: *Vertigo,* Dix M R and Hood J D (eds.) pp. 291–319. Chichester: John Wiley and Sons.

Luxon L M (1984) A bit dizzy. *British Journal of Hospital Medicine,* **32**(6): 315–321.

Pain

Armenian H K, Chamieh M A and Baraka A (1981) Influence of wartime stress and psychosocial factors in Lebanon on analgesic requirements for postoperative pain. *Social Science in Medicine,* **15E:** 63–66.

Blau J N (1983) Chronic headaches in general practice. *British Medical Journal,* **286**(1): 1375–1376.

Broome A K (1984) Psychological approaches to chronic pain. *Nursing Times,* **80**(6): 36–39.

Crow R and Hayward J (1979) Chronic pain. *Nursing,* 1st Series, **2**(2): 56.

Fordham M (1986) Neurophysiological pain theories. *Nursing*, 3rd Series, **3**(10): 365–372.

Gallop S M (1983) *Patient Teaching: Pain and Pain Control.* Edinburgh: Churchill Livingstone.

Lambley P (1980) *The Headache Book: A Self-Help Guide for Headache and Migraine Sufferers.* London: W J Allen.

Melzack R and Wall P D (1982) *The Challenge of Pain.* Harmondsworth: Penguin.

Osmond H, Mullaly R and Bisbee C (1984) The pain of depression compared with physical pain. *The Practitioner*, **228**(1395): 849–853.

Porter D, Leviton A, Slack W V and Graham J R (1981) A headache chronicle: the daily recording of headaches and their correlates. *Journal of Chronic Diseases*, **34**, 481–486.

Rose F C and Gawel M (1979) *Migraine: The Facts.* Oxford: Oxford University Press.

Speculand B, Goss A N, Spence N D and Pilowsky I (1981) Intractable facial pain and illness behaviour. *Pain*, **11**(2): 213–219.

Wilkinson M (1982) *Migraine and Headaches: Understanding, Controlling and Avoiding the Pain.* London: Martin Dunitz.

Dysphagia

Axelsson K, Norberg A and Asplund K (1986) Relearning to eat late after a stroke by systematic nursing intervention. *Journal of Advanced Nursing*, **11**(5): 553–559.

Cockcroft G and Ray M (1985) Feeding problems in stroke patients. *Nursing Mirror*, **160**(9): 26–29.

Hargrove R (1980) Feeding the severely dysphagic patient. *Journal of Neurosurgical Nursing*, **12**(2): 102–107.

Lavers A (1982) Feeding difficulties in patients with Huntington's chorea. *Nursing Times*, **78**(22): 920–921.

Sexuality

Webb C (1985) Teaching sexuality in the curriculum. *Senior Nurse*, **3**(5): 10–12.

Chapter 3

THE NURSE'S CORE INFORMATION

Chapter theme

To cope with any illness, it is essential to have a knowledge of the facts. The certainty of something bad is more bearable than uncertainty of any kind. Many people are relieved to find that their symptoms are medically recognisable and are neither imagined nor due to some psychological disorder. On learning that they have a specific disease people are usually keen to discover all that they can about it, to make their own decisions and control their treatment. Patients often derive considerable benefit from becoming an expert on their own medical condition.

When talking to a recently diagnosed patient it is necessary to replace fear of the unknown with an understanding of the disease and its effects. The skill of knowing when the questioner really wants factual information and when emotional support is required may depend more on the nurse's experience of talking to patients, her emotional maturity and her sensitivity than on any technique that can be taught formally. Armed with the knowledge of what can be done about his condition and what is likely to happen in the future, the patient will be able to make the best possible plans and arrangements.

The nurse who wishes to investigate a symptom will find in this chapter information on the course of disease, significant symptoms and the physiological changes involved in neurological illness. As there is much ignorance and misunderstanding about *the epilepsies*, this section is more detailed than the others.

Contents

Cerebrovascular accidents (CVAs)

Stroke

The word 'stroke' is generally accepted to mean a sudden ischaemic or haemorrhagic episode in the brain, which often results in some focal neurological deficit, most usually paralysis. The word 'stroke' suggests a blow that is sudden and complete. For the victim it is a catastrophic event. It comes out of the blue, with little or no warning, to alter dramatically a way of living. A few people recover with no disability but many more, if they survive the initial stroke, are left with some degree of incapacity. The scale of the problem in human terms is very great. There is an increasing incidence with age, but almost one-quarter of all cerebrovascular accident victims are under the age of 65 years (Lishman, 1987). Survivors of CVA constitute a large proportion of the severely disabled in Western societies. A major stroke can cause loss of consciousness, aphasia, hemiplegia, visual deficits, dysarthria and body image problems. (See Chapter 5, 'Russell'.)

Atheroma

A blood vessel may be narrowed by the accumulation of fatty tissue formed in the inner wall of the artery. This is known as atheroma or atherosclerosis. The fatty deposits gradually increase in size and become covered with connective tissue, forming a constriction that impedes and impairs the circulation.

Ischaemia

The term *ischaemia* means shortage of blood supply. Attacks indicating ischaemia in the distribution of one carotid artery are often referred to as episodes of carotid insufficiency. Those involving the brain stem are described as vertebrobasilar insufficiency because the vertebral and basilar arteries are involved.

Transient ischaemic attacks (TIAs)

A transient ischaemic attack is a temporary sudden episode of neurological disturbance, such as blurred or double vision, of presumed vascular origin, which typically lasts for only a few minutes. A complete recovery follows within 24 hours. 'Pieces of a clot break off and are carried by the blood stream, but instead of blocking an artery inside the brain completely, do so for a few moments only, then break off and pass on through the circulation so that normal blood supply is restored' (Bickerstaff, 1987). The episodes may be isolated and infrequent or may occur many times in a day and they tend to be consistent in each individual.

Where one person always has a visual blackout, another sees two of everything, i.e. diplopia, and yet another has vertigo, and most people will have at least two of these symptoms simultaneously.

TIAs in the posterior circulation can give rise to many symptoms:

- double vision, hemianopia, vertigo, ataxia (loss of muscular coordination when walking);
- paraesthesia (pins and needles) around the mouth, dysphagia and dysarthria;
- numbness or weakness of one half of the body or of all of the limbs.

Transient ischaemic attacks are regarded as a sign of an impending stroke. (See Chapter 5, 'Quentin' and 'Oliver'.)

Cerebral embolism

A small clot of fibrin or fat or a bubble of air carried in the blood stream may be too big to pass through a vessel in the brain, obstructing it by becoming lodged in the artery. Usually the patient has one large embolus and many smaller emboli. The clinical manifestations depend on the duration of the obstruction, the situation and extent of the ischaemic area and the adequacy of collateral circulation in providing an alternative route.

Cerebral thrombosis or thrombus

A clot on the damaged and roughened lining of an arteriosclerotic artery may suddenly block the blood supply to the brain. Most patients with cerebral thrombosis have arteriosclerotic disease affecting the cerebral arteries. All major arteries can be involved, but there is a predilection for the coronary and cerebral arteries. The arteriosclerotic plaques tend to be found at points of great mechanical stress in the vascular tree, e.g., where vessels branch.

Brain-stem stroke

Lesions in the vertebrobasilar arteries cause brain-stem strokes. These can be problematic as there are many different neural pathways passing through this region. Vital functions can be affected because of disturbance to the fibres serving the respiratory and cardiac centres. There may be loss of consciousness, and dysphagia due to bulbar weakness, increasing the risk of aspiration (inhalation of food).

Cerebral infarction

Cerebral infarction signifies blockage of a cerebral artery by thrombosis or embolism and the death of brain tissue. The blockage of an artery anywhere in the body results in death of the segment of tissue supplied by that artery. The brain is more sensitive than any other organ to a reduction in or cessation of blood flow because, once damaged, brain tissue cannot be replaced and because it also requires a constant supply of oxygen, enzymes and glucose to function. The brain damage resulting from cerebral infarction depends upon:

- the territory supplied by the artery;
- the actual site of the blockage;
- the potential collateral supply from adjacent vessels.

Cerebral haemorrhage

Intracerebral haemorrhage may be due to rupture of small penetrating arteries deep in the cerebral substance or secondary to abnormalities of blood vessels. These include arteriovenous malformations and congenital cerebral aneurysms. Congenital aneurysms tend to bleed into the subarachnoid space but there may be intracerebral spread of the haemorrhage.

Angiomas

Another cause of cerebral haemorrhage is associated with cerebral *arteriovenous malformation* or *angiomas*. Many such lesions remain asymptomatic throughout the patient's life. In many cases focal epilepsy is the main problem, while in others recurrent subarachnoid haemorrhage occurs with good recovery between attacks. This is because the haemorrhage is from blood vessels under low pressure, lacking the destructive power of a jet of arterial blood from a ruptured aneurysm or artery.

Subarachnoid haemorrhage

A subarachnoid haemorrhage is defined as bleeding into the cranial subarachnoid space. This may be due to head injury, an intracerebral haemorrhage, the rupture of an abnormality of the blood vessels or an aneurysm. The commonest cause is a cerebral aneurysm on the Circle of Willis and subarachnoid haemorrhage occurs most commonly after the age of 40. Less than 15 per cent of patients have symptoms prior to rupture and these usually consist of episodes of sudden headache, nausea, vomiting and neck stiffness. The diagnosis is made from the clinical history and a CT scan. Angiography is performed within the first 2 weeks as preparation for surgery. Those patients who have extensive central nervous system damage may not be suitable candidates for surgery, although this is the preferred treatment. There is a significant risk of re-bleeding, particularly in the weeks after the first haemorrhage.

Treatment of cerebrovascular accidents

The medical care of patients with cerebrovascular disease varies depending upon the age and condition of the patient and the doctor's preferences. Elderly patients admitted to a geriatric unit are mobilised early if their condition allows. Younger patients tend to be treated more conservatively, i.e. with a longer period of bedrest.

When patients are cared for in hospital the aim of the nursing staff is to teach them to become as independent as possible, so ensuring that their rehabilitation is a full-time activity. The nurse will be involved in all aspects of personal care. All treatments started in physiotherapy and other departments should be supported and continued in the ward. The patient should be encouraged to be as independent as possible; therefore, the amount of assistance given by the nurse should be the minimum required in order to allow the basic activities of life to take place. It is better that the disadvantage of slowness should be accepted in allowing patients to do things for themselves rather than all activities being done by, or fully assisted by, nurses. Sometimes allowing patients to do these activities unaided involves a specific risk but this may have to be accepted. This is partly in order to allow staff to assess accurately ability and safety levels and partly to encourage the development of independence. It is most important to prevent patients from becoming helpless and passive dependants.

Drugs such as hypotensive agents may be used where appropriate. Surgical treatment is aimed mainly at those patients with intracranial aneurysms and arteriovenous malformations. Patients with transient ischaemic attacks may be prevented from developing a complete stroke by aspirin or anticoagulant therapy. Surgical treatment may be by means of carotid endarterectomy if atheroma is causing carotid stenosis.

Degenerative disorders

Multiple sclerosis

The clinical course of multiple sclerosis varies remarkably from patient to patient. It can be remitting, progressive and remitting by turns, or progressive from the onset. After one or more isolated lesions have caused local symptoms, such as a sudden weakness in one or both legs or visual symptoms for a few days or weeks, there is usually a long remission period of months or even years. (See Chapter 5, 'Monica'.) The next attack may affect the same or other areas and fresh signs may appear, such as slight frequency of micturition, paraesthesia (pins and needles) or a feeling of heaviness in one leg, which tends to drag a little. In most patients the legs become most affected.

It is almost impossible to forecast how any given individual will be affected by multiple sclerosis; because the disease has a naturally variable course, patients may only attend hospital when they relapse and there may be no connection between disease activity and disability. The minority of patients who have acute multiple sclerosis experience a rapid onset of severe, often devastating disability (See Chapter 5, 'Nora'), while those with a benign form of the disease enjoy a normal life span with few, if any, symptoms or signs. Each patient usually has a mixture of symptoms, such as jerky spastic movements in the legs, weakness and incoordination of arm movements and lack of postural stability of the trunk and proximal limb joints. The symptoms are separated in time (*disseminated*) as well as in place (*plaques of demyelination forming at varying sites*), so that there are periods when the patient experiences symptoms while at other times he is in remission and is less troubled by the disorder.

The optic nerve and optic chiasma are often involved early in the course of the disease and blurring of vision, soon reduced to near blindness, may be the symptom that causes most patients to seek medical advice. When the patient visits his doctor complaining of visual symptoms he will describe a darkening or grey cloud over the centre of the visual field, which slowly becomes more opaque over a few days.

The period of visual deterioration varies considerably from person to person. Between 15 and 50 per cent of patients who have visual problems (*retrobulbar neuritis*) may go on to get other manifestations of multiple sclerosis. A full symptomatic recovery is to be expected in 75 per cent of the patients with unilateral optic neuritis (Russell, 1983). (See Chapter 5, 'Monica', 'Forsythe' and 'Nora'.)

Physiology

Multiple sclerosis is a chronic disease affecting the white matter of the brain and spinal cord. Sometimes, it spreads into the grey matter of the cerebral cortex and in the cranial and spinal nerve roots. Small patches develop in which the myelin of the nerve fibres is destroyed and the axons become thinner than normal or disappear. The effect is either to destroy the nerve fibres or to interfere seriously with the transmission of impulses along the fibres in the central nervous system. Signs and symptoms vary according to the location of the plaques. If there are only small isolated patches, the symptoms arising from these focal lesions may gradually disappear as the patches shrink and other nerve fibres may take over the work of those that are damaged.

If, however, the disease progresses and more plaques develop, symptoms persist and get worse with increasing 'attacks' of demyelination. When the condition is advanced and symptoms have become stable the individual characteristics will depend upon where most of the sclerotic patches are in the nervous system. If the lesions are mainly in the cerebellar system, ataxia and hypertonic muscles will be the main problem. If the posterior column of the spinal cord is the most involved, there will be sensory ataxia and loss of postural sense, and sometimes a loss of the sense of touch. Extensive research programmes throughout the world have not identified the cause of plaque formation nor why it happens in certain individuals.

Mythology

Myths are more commonly associated with an illness such as multiple sclerosis that is both difficult to diagnose and has no established treatment. Unfortunately, the popular concept of multiple sclerosis is that all patients will end up in a wheelchair. In hospital, our view of multiple sclerosis is distorted since we tend to see the most severely affected individuals. In fact, less than 10 per cent of patients with multiple sclerosis will require wheelchair care. Many years may pass before there is a further attack – up to 20 years is not unusual. Many patients lead a normal life with minimal disability and the general rule is that patients recover from an acute attack. In the majority of patients control or containment of the disease process is irregular and intermittent. The patient's emotional reactions, intellectual understanding and capability of making an adjustment to the illness have a strong influence over the course of the disease (Rose, 1979).

Treatment

No treatment has been shown to control or cure the disease, although steroids do slow the progress of optic neuritis. Immunotherapy, special diets, interferons, penicillamine and hyperbaric oxygen have all been tried. However, the small numbers involved, lack of controls, short follow-up periods, non-randomised samples and highly selected populations limit the usefulness of such studies. Patients have tried many different diets including fish oil, linoleic acid, evening primrose oil and the gluten-free diets. Patients using hyperbaric oxygen (HBO) treatment breathe oxygen under increased pressure in a specially constructed chamber with controlled temperature and humidity. After 90 minutes the chamber is decompressed over a 10-minute period. A carefully conducted trial of this approach for 84 patients led to the conclusion that 'There appears to be little basis for recommending this treatment to patients with multiple sclerosis' (Wiles et al, 1986). The most recent attempts to find effective treatment include trials of total lymphoid irradiation, where the patient is irradiated every day for 2 weeks and their progress compared with patients who attend for radiotherapy but do not receive it.

Exercising and strengthening muscles, as well as medication, can reduce spasticity. Pain caused by optic neuritis can be relieved by steroids, while the pain of trigeminal neuralgia can usually be helped by Tegretol. The depressed patient will benefit from antidepressant therapy. After assessment of bladder function the patient may need to use an antispasmodic drug, regular catheterisation or an indwelling catheter. Constipation is helped by taking as much physical exercise as possible and increasing the amount of fruit, vegetables, bran and fluid in the diet.

Huntington's chorea

Stevens (1982) defines features of the disease: 'A neurological disorder which affects males and females equally and in the majority of patients, is characterised clinically by progressive chorea and dementia with onset in adult life. It is an inherited condition, the mode of transmission being autosomal dominance'. In discussing the natural history of the disorder, Stevens identifies 42 years as the average age of onset and the average duration of life after the onset of symptoms being about 14 years. Overall, he says, '90% are dead in twenty years. The mean age of death is about fifty-six years'.

People close to the patient may have noticed subtle mental changes that have occurred in their relative, with irritability, moodiness and impulsiveness, as well as depression, leading to a change in personality. Hayden (1981) explains that there may be obvious disturbances of functional ability in the early stages of the disease: 'The housewife may find that she is less able to look after the home and the businessman may find it more difficult to maintain his appointments and manage his financial affairs'.

The single most common complaint according to Hayden (1981) is jerkiness, clumsiness or mild incoordination, which usually heralds the onset of chorea. Initially:

The chorea may be minimal, but as the disease progresses the patient will be seen with ceaseless writhing, jerking and twisting of different parts of the body as a result of the interruption of the voluntary by involuntary movements. In some persons chorea may mainly affect the face, whilst in others the extremities will predominantly exhibit the hyperkinesia. When sitting at ease many patients show constant irregular motion of the hands and legs. The legs may be alternately crossed and uncrossed. Fingers are constantly flexed and extended and these movements are exaggerated when the patient holds his hands before him.

Nurses who have seen patients with Huntington's chorea will usually be able to recognise the distinctive afflictions that the disease imposes on sufferers. Most affected people stand on a broad base and no involuntary movements are to be seen. However, as soon as they begin to walk they become unsteady and sway about, with several false starts, and may fall. Their sideways movements appear to follow a 'zig-zagging' route. Unfortunately, this precarious gait has resulted in patients being presumed drunk. Injuries from falls are common and in many instances patients are unable to walk without assistance. Involuntary facial gestures, including pouting of the lips, twitching cheeks and elevation of the eyebrows, all draw attention to the restless agony imposed by Huntington's chorea.

The choreic symptoms may precede or follow the development of psychotic symptoms or mental deterioration. The impairment of complex facial movements gives way to constant grimacing. It no longer becomes possible to blow out the cheeks, display the teeth or to whistle. Nystagmus and difficulty in focusing are sometimes apparent. Difficulty with chewing and swallowing is often experienced, combined with excessive salivation. Involuntary movements make eating a frustrating experience for both patient and carer alike. (See Chapter 2, 'Dysphagia'.)

As the disease progresses, depression or manic moods, explosiveness and hypersensitivity may lead the patient to become withdrawn and apathetic. Auditory or visual hallucinations may occur. Emotional problems can lead to drug abuse, depression and suicide. With the onset of dementia, mentation problems become apparent in daily situations. The patient has difficulty in following the gist of a conversation; he becomes vague and uncertain in speech and fails to appreciate humour or subtle distinctions of meaning. One woman was observed by her husband to speak vaguely and off the point, to be repetitive and difficult to follow in her conversation, which was a notable change in someone who had had an academic career. One woman was thought by her family to have 'aged very remarkably' in a few months, with premature greying and skin changes such as wrinkling. Over time, earlier problems may be intensified, marriages sometimes collapse and if there are children a conflict of loyalties arises. In the terminal stages of the illness the patient will be a physical burden to nurse and the family may no longer be able to be the main carers; institutional help may be sought. (See Chapter 4, 'Feelings'.)

Physiology

Biochemical research during the last decade has shown that several different types of neurones die prematurely in the brains of patients with Huntington's chorea. The disease affects two main parts of the nervous system – the centres controlling bodily movements and some of the centres responsible for mental functions – so that both these functions may be disturbed. (See Chapter 5, 'Osbert'.)

Treatment

Drugs are given to patients with Huntington's chorea to reduce involuntary movements, treat behavioural disturbances or lift depression. As the chemical messenger in the brain is overactive and producing too much dopamine, a dopamine-depleting drug such as tetrabenazine (Nitoman) is used to treat involuntary movements. Dopamine receptor blockers include haloperidol (Serenace), pimozide (Orap) and sulpiride (Dolmatil), which diminish choreiform movements and alleviate behavioural problems. Benzodiazepines such as diazepam (Valium) and chlordiazepoxide (Librium) help to reduce tension and suppress chorea in some patients. Antidepressants may also be used to treat depression. Any of these drugs may interact with alcohol, so that a single measure may have an impact equivalent to a double or triple.

Motor neurone disease

Motor neurone disease is characterised by progressive weakness and muscular atrophy and most frequently develops between the ages of 40 and 60 years. The initial symptoms may be those of symmetrical spastic weakness of the legs, shoulders or neck muscles. The hand and shoulder girdle muscles begin to waste. Gradually the weakness and wasting spreads through the body and the trunk muscles no longer give support. Weakness of the tongue and throat muscles makes speech difficult and swallowing impossible. (See Chapter 4, 'Feelings'.)

Weight loss and easy fatiguing can greatly worry patients. Severe falls (defined as resulting in fractures or cuts needing stitches) are a common hazard, especially in more mobile people. Many patients with motor neurone disease suffer from painful cramps and in some these are nocturnal. Thirty-one per cent of one sample of patients who were investigated had poor sleep patterns. Other researchers have observed that patients with the disease experience minor aches and pains during the night from an inability to move normally, and the cumulative effect may be interruption of sleep (Norris et al, 1985). Because of lack of daily physical activity, and of abdominal muscle power to empty the rectum, constipation becomes an increasing problem, sometimes requiring manual evacuation. This is disturbing for close family members and should ideally be done by professional carers.

In a study of the symptoms of 42 patients with motor neurone disease Newrick and Langton-Hewer (1984) found that 'Pain, falls, constipation and swelling of the legs emerged as the major symptomatic problems. Two thirds of the patients appeared to be in need of aids which had not been provided.' The authors also explain that poor sleeping was due to a 'combination of worry, discomfort and secretions pooling in the throat (causing choking and drooling)'.

The survival rate is very low, the natural history being of decline and death from 1 to 15 years after the diagnosis has been confirmed. The prognosis is determined by the age of onset. In contrast to other diseases the prognosis is worst when the onset occurs in an older person than it would be starting in youth. Young patients experience more spasticity, dysarthria and develop a slow, stiff rolling gait. Older patients suffer from weakness, which, combined with peripheral nerve problems, could mean that they are considerably disabled.

Physiology

Motor neurones control striated voluntary muscle. Lower motor neurones occur at the spinal cord level and directly innervate the muscle. Upper motor neurones are the 'command neurones' located in the brain and influence the activity of lower motor neurones. In healthy people these neurones receive instructions from the brain and then send commands to contract to the appropriate muscle but in motor neurone disease this vital link between brain and muscle is lost. The abnormalities found differ according to whether the damage affects the upper or lower motor neurones: either may dominate the clinical picture but more often the signs are of a combined lesion. Although the brain is unaffected and the muscle cells are healthy, limb movements become difficult and eventually cease. The muscles of the chest wall may be similarly cut off, as may the muscles concerned with chewing and swallowing. The cause of the premature death of neurones is unknown. Unlike in Parkinson's disease, there is no drug treatment that can partially compensate for the loss of motor neurones.

Treatment

By careful symptom control the quality of life can be improved. Ideally, the patient is cared for wherever he would like to be but he needs to know that when he is dying help will be available. Whether he attends a day centre, spends short periods in a hospice or remains at home, team support is necessary, with one designated key worker to coordinate the activities of different professionals. The patient needs time to communicate his needs. When speech is affected it is important for the nurse to remember that the patient's intellect is not impaired, nor is he deaf or foreign: by listening to him the nurse can assess his physical, emotional, social and spiritual needs. An important aim of treatment is to anticipate crisis and avoid it rather than reacting to, say, a choking incident. Physiotherapy will be needed to maximise muscle power, prevent joint stiffness, maintain chest expansion and assist coughing.

Pain can be controlled by diamorphine to suppress coughing and alleviate the distress. Dysphagia can be avoided by careful feeding and administration of atropine sulphate and antidepressants. Early intervention for dysphagia by the speech therapist enables the carer to develop alternative feeding methods. Speech therapy and aids to attract attention are needed by patients who have dysarthria. Muscle stiffness can be alleviated by correct positioning, physiotherapy and a benzodiazepine drug. The patient with insomnia may need better positioning and medication to control his pain.

Above all, the nurse must listen to the frustration, anger and guilt experienced by the patient and his family. A depressed patient may also need antidepressants. The complexity of the relationships between carers will affect the way people react to the death of the patient. The nurse may need to discuss with relatives and colleagues what went well, what went wrong and how they could have done things differently.

Movement disorders

Parkinson's disease

On hearing his name being called, the patient in the waiting room has difficulty initially in getting out of his chair, particularly if it has no arm rests. He stands stooped, appearing uncertain of how best to initiate walking, his feet appearing to stick to the floor. Tremor may be noted in one or both legs before the first step is taken. When walking begins the steps are small and shuffling. Once walking is under way, the typical 'festinant' gait is seen. The patient may almost break into a run as he tries to catch up with himself since his forward stoop pushes his centre of gravity further and further in front of him. On reaching the entrance to the consulting room he pauses, seemingly disturbed by his conception of the narrowness of the doorway and may stop altogether. The whole cycle is then repeated.

In the early stages of the disease the symptoms are a nuisance but constitute no disability or handicap – tremor that causes embarrassment or an awkwardness with fine movement making certain tasks slow and laborious. Chief among the signs and symptoms are a masklike face, speech difficulties, tremor, stooped posture and abnormalities of gait. The symptoms may develop bilaterally with minimum disability, whereas if a tremor was present initially only in one hand, it may later affect both. The patient begins to experience problems in getting about. Later, he may experience significant disability due to increasing slowness and poverty of movement (*akinesia*), rigidity and gait disturbance. In spite of its dramatic nature the tremor itself is less disabling than are the accompanying rigidity and akinesia. The symptoms produce a definite disability so that certain tasks have to be avoided altogether or can only be done at certain times of the day. Other symptoms that almost inevitably develop are increased sweating, undue sensitivity to heat, excessive salivation and emotional disturbance. Another common problem is *micrographia*, when the handwriting becomes progressively smaller and may trail away to nothing. The course of the disease is usually progressively chronic extending over one or more decades. The worst, and relatively rare, form of the disease means that the victim is dependent on his family or professional carers as mobility and self-caring skills may have been overtaken by its progress.

Physiology

The symptoms have been traced to widespread diffuse lesions in the basal ganglia. Although the degenerative changes are widespread, the basal nucleus, the substantia nigra, is severely affected, with almost complete loss of its melanin-containing cells. A decrease of dopamine in the substantia nigra is found. It is thought that the disturbance of the function of these cells and their eventual destruction results from this deficiency, for dopamine is essential to the transmission of nerve impulses in the basal ganglia.

Treatment

All the treatments for Parkinson's disease are aimed at altering neuronal function but do nothing to correct the underlying disease process, which remains progressive. The introduction of levodopa a quarter of a century ago, the development of dopamine agonists within the last decade, new imaging devices, e.g. magnetic resonance imaging (MRI) and positron emission tomography (PET), have all resulted in enthusiastic research projects being developed to pursue the cause and cure for the disorder.

Judicious and conservative use of anti-Parkinsonian medication in the early stages of the disease prolongs the usefulness of the drugs and doctors often rely on patients to report their observations on the effect of medications prescribed. The weaker anticholinergics are used first. Later, once the patient has become aware of the necessity for commitment to continuous treatment, it is time to begin levodopa therapy. Bromocriptine (Parlodel) protects against long-term side-effects of levodopa i.e. involuntary movements. Adapting to living with Parkinson's disease is largely dependent on the supportive networks of family, friends and work colleagues, as alterations may need to be made to the person's home and working life-style. A variety of professional therapists, e.g. occupational and speech therapists and community nurses, may also contribute.

Benign essential tremor

Benign essential tremor is often a familial disorder that may begin at any age. Patients come to the doctor because they are embarrassed or worried that people will think they have been drinking. The tremor is obvious when sustaining a posture and persists on movement but is completely abolished when the affected limb is at rest. At first, the tremor is only present at times of heightened tension, particularly when the individual is under observation in public. A gradual increase in severity over many years may mean that, eventually, handwriting, shaving or drinking from a cup will become difficult, even when at peace and alone. Frequently, there is a tremor of the head (*titubation*) or jaw, and the voice may sound tremulous. Alcohol temporarily alleviates this tremor. (See Chapter 5, 'Frank'.)

The dystonias

In this group of conditions sustained contractions of agonist and antagonist muscle groups result in abnormal (sometimes painful) postures. These may be associated with slow writhing movements of the affected parts, which may be present continually or only during specific motor acts. The condition may be confined to a few muscle groups affecting the use of the hand during writing (writer's cramp), causing spasmodic turning of the head and neck to one side (*spasmodic torticollis*) or closure of the eyes (*blepharospasm*), or it may be generalised, causing distorted body postures (See Chapter 5, 'Greta').

Different types of dystonia tend to affect different age groups (Table 3.1).

Table 3.1 *Dystonia and age*

Dystonia type	Age group affected
Spasmodic torticollis	30–40 years
Meige's syndrome	50-year-olds
Occupational cramp	People in their 30s

Spasmodic torticollis

The focal dystonia called torticollis has been defined as 'a condition in which there are repeated purposeless movements of the head and neck or sustained abnormal postures or both. There is always an element of spasm' (Tibbets, 1981). Men and women are equally affected and the typical age of onset is between 30 and 45 years. In spasmodic torticollis the neck tends to become twisted to one side by sustained intermittent spasms of the sternomastoid and other cervical muscles. Pain is a common feature of this condition and after some years serious changes of the cervical spine occur. A quarter of patients experience a natural remission. Historically, there has been much dispute about the cause – for the past two decades the emphasis has been on organic factors. (See Chapter 5, Linda.)

Occupational cramp

The occupational dystonias are a group of conditions characterised by the breakdown of a particular learned motor skill, essential for the normal execution of the affected individual's trade. Those people in occupations in which repetitive, intricate, finely co-ordinated hand and finger movements are demanded are particularly at risk (Lees, 1985).

When a concert pianist develops dystonia it is virtually untreatable in view of the virtuosity required to play his instrument at the highest level. Spasms of the finger muscles prevent rapid finger movements or a single finger may remain extended for a few seconds instead of striking the correct note; all the fingers may run together in staccato passages and some pianists have found the left forefinger constantly touching the keyboard. Typist's cramp may begin with loss of speed, pain in the fingers and involuntary flexing or extending of the little or ring fingers. The disorder may prevent the patient from being able to type at all.

Technological advances, increasing automation and shorter working hours have helped to eradicate many occupational dystonias, but typists, telegraphists, classical musicians and some groups of professional sportsmen may also be affected' (Lees, 1985).

Meige's syndrome

Most patients with Meige's syndrome initially complain of involuntary contractions of the eyelids (blepharospasm), followed by an inability to open them by the usual means because of sustained spasm of the orbicularis oculi and surrounding muscles. As the disorder progresses, involuntary eyelid closure interferes with an increasing number of the patient's daily activities. The eyelids may go into spasm on crossing the road, while at work or during leisure pursuits. Later, the patient has to hold his eyelids open with his fingers in order to see.

> Many patients become increasingly withdrawn and depressed as they find that any outside contact or pleasurable excitement increases the spasms. Indoor hobbies are also denied as reading, watching television or doing needlework may induce eyelid closure. The patient's daily activities become increasingly limited and he may eventually lose his job and social independence (Lees, 1985).

Rest is the most effective relieving factor and after a good night's sleep, blepharospasm often disappears for an hour or two in the early morning, which is the only time patients can do their daily chores before their eyes begin to close again. The patient has to be led around as if blind and loses normal eye contact with his loved ones.

> Depression tends to increase and the last few years of many patients' lives are spent in virtual total darkness with severe articulation, swallowing and breathing disabilities. Aspiration pneumonia and suicide are the two commonest disease related causes of death but most patients succumb to intercurrent illnesses (Lees, 1985).

Other facial movements may occur in the syndrome including chewing, lipsmacking and a darting protrusion of the tongue. (See Chapter 5, 'Joan' and 'Katya'.)

Treatment

Numerous drugs have been reported to be of benefit to some patients with torticollis. However, few drugs have given reliable relief and improvement occurs in only a minority of patients. Anticholinergic drugs such as benzhexol may be of value to about 20 per cent of patients but side-effects often restrict their uses. Botulinum toxin is a powerful presynaptic neurotoxin that inhibits release of acetylcholine. It has been used successfully to treat blepharospasm, hemifacial spasm and torticollis. Stell et al (1988) report: 'Botulinum toxin appears to be the most effective treatment for torticollis available at present.' The toxin is injected into the affected sternomastoid and posterior cervical muscles and successfully controls head position and pain in the majority of patients with torticollis. (See Chapter 5, 'Katya' and 'Linda'.)

Wilson's disease

In 1912 Kinnear Wilson defined a 'disease which is familial. It occurs in young people, either in an acute or chronic form.' This syndrome subsequently came to be known as Wilson's disease, in his honour. The findings he described include the gradual onset of tremor and muscular rigidity, which make walking, dressing, feeding and writing increasingly difficult. A characteristic of the disease is the flapping tremor, also termed wing-beating because it may be so forceful that it causes injury to the chest or abdomen. Eventually, the head and trunk can become involved in severe hyperkinetic movements. When the patient tries to eat, dress, write, wash or walk the intention tremor (i.e. a tremor that increases with deliberate movements) prevents normal activity, but this tremor is absent during sleep. Talking may be accompanied by a variety of facial grimaces, stereotyped gestures or rhythmic movements of the hands, feet or trunk, which appear to be helping the patient to articulate.

A graphic picture of a patient afflicted by Wilson's disease is provided by Scheinberg and Sternlieb (1984), who describe the consequent overwhelming frustration of a patient, 'who cannot talk, walk, eat or kiss, because his intellectual capacities and emotional sensitivities are generally little, if at all, diminished.' The state of dependency increases until the patient could die from respiratory or genitourinary infection or renal failure. Marsden (1987) explains that the symptoms of Wilson's disease 'usually appear between the ages of 5 and 50 years. In those who present with neurological abnormalities, the onset usually occurs in the second or third decade. The appearance of symptoms before adolescence, or after the age of 40 is unusual.'

Physiology

In normal infants the liver develops the ability to synthesise caeruloplasmin by 3 months of age, but in the child born with a genetic tendency to develop Wilson's disease, liver function never matures. Wilson's disease is a disorder of metabolism in which the blood protein caeruloplasmin, which normally transports copper in the blood, is deficient, copper cannot be excreted into the biliary system and excess copper accumulates in the body. Copper concentrations in the liver can be up to 20 times those of healthy subjects. As the disease progresses, the hepatic concentration increases until the patient develops obvious signs of liver failure. Clinical manifestations of the disease depend on the site and rate at which the excess copper is deposited in various organs, especially the liver and the brain.

Treatment

Since 1912 a clearer understanding of the disease has been advanced and the role of copper appreciated, so that effective forms of therapy have been developed and the course of the illness is no longer 'progressively and invariably fatal'. The introduction of penicillamine as a binding agent for the removal of copper has revolutionised the prognosis, so that no patient should now die of Wilson's disease provided it has been identified before severe and irreversible tissue damage has occurred. The main aim of treatment is to prevent further neurological damage. Lifelong treatment is necessary as the fundamental defect is part of the patient's genetic legacy and, as such, is not altered by treatment. Penicillamine slowly increases the urinary excretion of copper by removing the deposits in the brain and liver, which may produce a remarkable remission. The patient's improved state of health can be maintained for many years when treatment commences early in the disease, with only a minor biochemical disorder remaining, suggesting chronic active hepatitis or cirrhosis of the liver.

Gilles de la Tourette syndrome

This socially disabling condition is a cluster of symptoms that commonly occur together. It starts in childhood or adolescence, with generalised multiple tics and inappropriate vocalisations. Tics are abrupt, visually repetitive, coordinated muscular jerks. Lees et al (1984) reviewed 53 patients and concluded that the face was most commonly affected with eye-blinking and grimacing, followed by head movements, shoulder shrugs, arm jerks and neck tics. Trimble (1983) explained that 'Some abnormal facial movements are seen in almost all patients, while involvement of the lower limbs and trunk is less frequent.' Lees et al (1984) identified many of their patients who had a 'virtually limitless repertoire of abnormal movements which had waxed and waned throughout childhood and adolescence'.

Lees et al also found that compulsive touching was present in 61 per cent of their 53 patients. Popular objects to touch included hot things, such as fires and lighted cigarettes, door handles, railings and floors. Compulsive touching of breasts, bottoms and hair was also frequent. Striking was usually directed towards the patient's own body and was commoner in females. One patient gouged his eye badly by constant picking and scratching and another detached his retina as a consequence of repeated blows to the head.

Lawden's (1986) literature review revealed that 'abnormal vocalizations are eventually produced by all patients with the Tourette syndrome'. These could be meaningless grunts, barks, hisses or whistles or the production of formed words. Tics and vocalisations, according to Lees et al (1984), are invariably aggravated by anxiety, stress or excitement, but other occasional provoking factors include fatigue, boredom, talking to strangers, watching television, derogatory personal comments addressed to the patient and depression. Sleep, relaxation or concentration or an enjoyable task usually lead to their temporary disappearance and some people have identified music, driving a motor vehicle, dancing, agreeable company, alcohol and love-making as activities that reduce the tics.

Lawden (1986) goes on to report that:

The disease is not truly progressive, but pursues a fluctuating course throughout the patient's life. Complete remissions are rare, but the symptoms change over a period of months, both in severity and in the groups of muscles affected. Patients are usually able to suppress their symptoms for short periods, though this may be terminated by an explosive outburst.

The forced utterance of single obscenities (*coprolalia*) spontaneously disappears in about one-third of patients later in life, although other features of the disease rarely remit. (See Chapter 5, 'Hanna', 'Harry' and 'Isaac'.)

Physiology

Opinion has long been divided over whether symptoms of the Tourette syndrome derive from organic neurological disease or from psychological factors. Lawden (1986) points to evidence which 'suggests that decreasing dopaminergic transmission relieves Tourette symptoms'. He also explains that different drugs are effective for motor and behavioural features of the disease: 'So perhaps they may have their basis in different transmitter systems'. Evidence to support the organic argument about the syndrome is also found in the high male:female sex ratio, genetic factors and the stereotyped clinical picture. It is also known that tics and vocalisations may occasionally be acquired following encephalitis, a head injury or carbon monoxide poisoning. Coprolalia can occur as a result of structural damage to the central nervous system and occasionally patients with severe aphasia following a stroke may still utter obscenities.

Treatment

Lawden (1986) reports that haloperidol was found to eliminate or reduce symptoms in 80–89 per cent of cases in his study. When the sedation and drug-induced movements produced by this drug are intolerable other neuroleptics such as pimozide may produce fewer side-effects. Clonidine is more effective in treating behavioural aspects of the condition than in tic control. In a 24-year-old man who said his main problem was his 'nerves', the tension and strain produced by the disorder, with embarrassing head thrusts and vocal grunts, was successfully treated with clonidine, which made him feel calmer.

The epilepsies

Epileptic seizures are generally believed to be due to an abnormal electrical discharge by nerve cells within the brain. As there are many different forms of epilepsy it is important for the nurse to understand which type of disorder the individual patient experiences so that she can make an important contribution towards his education. In learning about his condition the patient develops a realistic view of how epilepsy affects him, rather than adopting the simplified, stigmatising identity of an epileptic.

Primary generalised

In many instances of epilepsy there is no evident anatomical pathology and the occurrence of seizures is the sole manifestation of a constitutionally determined low seizure threshold. Everyone has an inborn tendency to have an epileptic attack and in some people their low seizure threshold causes epilepsy.

Symptomatic

Any injury or disorder affecting a part of the brain may produce a scar or epileptic focus, which subsequently triggers epileptic seizures (Table 3.2). The focus may be caused by a head injury, perhaps at birth or as a result of a motor accident, or by meningitis. Post-traumatic epilepsy may follow serious injury to the brain, particularly if an injury has penetrated the dura mater and brain. If there was no loss of consciousness or skull fracture at the time of the injury, the onset of epilepsy is very rare.

Classification of seizures

In the international classification of epilepsy, seizures are named by manner and location of onset. Some partial or focal seizures begin in a single area of the brain while others have a generalised onset. The clinical manifestation or change in behaviour that takes place is dependent on the specific area of the brain where the abnormal electrical discharge is occurring at any particular moment.

Partial seizures (begin in a local or focal area)

Simple—no impairment of consciousness
    With motor symptoms
    With sensory symptoms
    With autonomic symptoms
    Compound forms

Table 3.2   *Causes and ages of epilepsy*

New born	Child	Adult
Birth trauma	Fever	Idiopathic
Meningitis	Idiopathic	Stroke
Hypoglycaemia	Abscess	Head injury
Hypocalcaemia	Head injury	Abscess
	Congenital	Systemic disease
	Tuberose sclerosis	Infection
	Infection	Encephalitis
	Encephalitis	Meningitis
	Meningitis	Tumours
	Tumours	

Complex—consciousness impaired
  Impairment of consciousness only
  With cognitive symptoms
  With affective symptoms
  With psychosensory symptoms
  With psychomotor symptoms
  Compound forms

Generalised seizures

  Absences (formerly called *petit mal*)
  Myoclonic seizures
  Clonic seizures
  Tonic seizures
  Tonic-clonic seizures (formerly called *grand mal*)
  Atonic seizures

Partial (focal) seizures

These can occur without any impairment of consciousness, depending upon the anatomical site or origin of the seizure discharge: motor, sensory or autonomic. A partial seizure can evolve to become secondarily generalised, producing a tonic-clonic (formerly called *grand mal*) convulsion. A generalised seizure occurs when disturbance of electrical activity affects the whole of both hemispheres of the brain, producing absences, myoclonic, clonic, tonic, tonic-clonic, major convulsive and atonic seizures.

Complex partial

The part of the brain involved varies from patient to patient but the focus is generally in the temporal lobe. The electrical discharge in the brain during the attack may spread slowly and without causing a convulsion. Seizures originating in the temporal lobe cause complex disorders of sensation, the most frequent at the beginning of an attack being a curious feeling that starts in the pit of the stomach and rises towards the throat. The hallucinations may be of simple sensory phenomena such as odours or single sounds or may consist of highly-developed psychic disturbances. The abnormal discharge may sometimes merely cause a sudden disturbance of behaviour. The gustatory and olfactory hallucinations are usually rather unpleasant and may be accompanied by chewing movements and smacking of the lips.

    Two transient memory disturbances are characteristic of seizures originating in the temporal lobe: jamais vu and déjà vu. Jamais vu is a sudden feeling of unfamiliarity while the patient is in his own environment. Déjà vu is a vivid sense of familiarity with the current situation. Although the experience may be quite new to the individual, he feels that 'It has all happened before', 'I have been here before'. The time scale of memory is disordered so that events are interpreted out of sequence. During the attack the patient may not fall but is in a dreamy state, during which he may continue with his normal activity. There may be a complete amnesia for these events after the attack. Normal behaviour is usually resumed over a matter of minutes.

Patients often have difficulty describing what happens in a complex partial seizure because of the intangible quality of their subjective symptoms and they may say, 'It was just a sour taste in my mouth – a burning sour taste', 'It just feels like something is coming through my head', 'There is a sensation that the top of my mouth drops down to the bottom'.

Generalised seizures

Secondarily generalised.   Any seizure discharge beginning in one focal area of the brain, for example, the temporal lobe, can start as a feeling of déjà vu and then change into a partial complex seizure with a lapse or impairment of consciousness. Chadwick and Usiskin (1987) explain that 'One characteristic of the electrical discharge at the basis of seizures is its tendency to spread from the site of onset to other parts of the brain'. If the seizure discharge spreads out to the rest of the brain, the person can have a generalised tonic-clonic fit.

Absences.   The *absence* (formerly known as petit mal) is the simplest and briefest kind of fit: it usually occurs without warning and has no recovery stage. This type of attack is merely a brief lapse of full consciousness, sometimes accompanied by rhythmical blinking of the eyelids. The patient's awareness of his surroundings is altered – he never knows quite where he is or what is happening. Recovery is immediate and there are no sequelae. These small attacks are most frequent in the morning on rising, although there may be many hundreds throughout the course of the day, which can seriously interfere with education. Absence seizures begin to occur in childhood and adolescence and only occasionally persist into adult life.

Myoclonus.   Myoclonus is a form of primary generalised epilepsy that develops in early childhood and manifests as a shock-like jerking of the muscles. This may happen in the arms, especially first thing in the morning, and it sometimes occurs without other signs of epilepsy. Similar jerks on dropping off to sleep occur in normally healthy people. Various types of generalised fits occur, including sudden jerking movements of the limbs.

Tonic-clonic.   During the days or hours before an attack the patient may experience feelings of irritability and various minor disturbances such as myoclonic jerks. The onset of the actual fit is sudden. There may be a momentary feeling of strangeness (the *aura*) but almost immediately the patient is struck unconscious and falls rigid to the ground; this is the tonic phase, characterised by powerful muscular contraction. Air is forced from the chest, sometimes in a loud cry, and the teeth are clenched. No respiratory movements occur and the patient becomes cyanosed.

The tonic phase lasts for about half a minute and is followed by the clonic phase. This consists of violent convulsive movements of the limbs, which occur with gradually decreasing frequency. The lips, tongue or cheek may be bitten. The combination of relaxed sphincters and the contraction of the abdominal musculature may cause voiding of urine and, less often, of faeces.

The clonic phase is followed by a complete relaxation of the muscles, when the patient will sleep or rouse gradually. The period of unconsciousness generally lasts for a few minutes, during which time the pupils are large and unreacting. On recovering consciousness the patient is likely to be confused and may complain of headache, nausea and drowsiness.

Atonic.   Atonic seizures occur when the patient suddenly loses muscle tone in his legs and drops to the ground. He may injure himself but, if not, within 10 seconds to 1 minute later he will get up and go about his business without any ill-effects.

Status epilepticus.   The condition of status epilepticus exists when repeated epileptic seizures occur without recovery. In the case of generalised convulsive status epilepticus, prompt treatment, which may take the form of intravenous medication, is required to maintain life.

First aid in epilepsy

DO
Try to move away any objects that might be a danger to the patient having the attack. Only consider moving the patient if this is impossible. Lie the patient down in the recovery position, usually on the floor or ground, and loosen any tight clothing. Stay with the patient until he recovers consciousness, if necessary until arrangements have been made to escort him home. Nurses may need to record observed fits for ward or medical use. If someone is having a succession of fits without regaining consciousness between them, i.e. status epilepticus, call a doctor immediately. As nonconvulsive fits take many forms, the response of observers will need to vary. If a patient falls abruptly, it is necessary to ensure that he has not sustained any injury that requires attention. If prolonged confusion occurs, gently protect the patient from obvious dangers (like wandering into the road) and keep other people from crowding round. Stay with the patient until he is able to resume his normal routine or find his own way home.

DO NOT
Attempt to restrain the convulsive movements. In particular, do not put anything in the patient's mouth in an attempt to prevent him from biting his tongue. Do not give anything to drink until the patient is fully awake. If recovery is speedy and uncomplicated, there is no need to summon medical help.

Information needs

When people feel that nurses and doctors give them insufficient information about epilepsy they will turn to other sources, thus indicating a failure to provide a good nursing service. The nurse has a responsibility to identify and meet information needs of her patients. Questions on how to identify attitudes towards epilepsy were provided in Chapter 1 and factual information is discussed here. Nurses who talk to patients can sometimes offer practical advice; at other times they will learn from their patients about living with epilepsy.

Seizures

A non-intrusive way of assessing a patient's needs is to enquire about the information needed by people who have epilepsy. Specific topics may need discussion such as the type of seizure disorder, the patient's understanding of the cause of seizures, the place of electroencephalography (EEG) and anything that exacerbates the seizures, such as missing meals, losing sleep or an increase in emotional pressures.

Treatment

The nurse has to pay particular attention to medication because of the consequences of non-compliance or drug interaction. To identify information needs she can enquire whether or not the patient sees any benefit from taking his medication and knows what would happen if he stopped. Perhaps he has had a bad experience related to taking tablets and would benefit from additional information about how to take them and how often (Table 3.3) and side-effects or interactions with other drugs. The patient may need to be informed about exemption from prescription charges.

Table 3.3 *Anticonvulsant therapy*

First line drugs	Second line drugs

Phenytoin (Epanutin)
    Average daily dose 200–400 mg
	Clonazempam (Rivotril)
	    Average daily dose range 1–3 mg, twice daily

Carbamazepine (Tegretol)
    Average daily dose range 600–1200 mg, two or three times daily
	Clobazam (Frisium)
	    Average daily dose range 10–30 mg, once daily

Sodium valproate (Epilium)
    Average daily dose 600–1500 mg, once or twice daily
	Primidone (Mysoline)
	    Average daily dose range (adults) 500-1000 mg, twice daily

Ethosuximide (Zarontin)
    Average daily dose 500–1000 mg on mg/ kg basis, 2 or 3 times daily
	Phenobarbitone
	    Average daily dose (adults) 60–120 mg, once or twice daily

Fear

Most social impairments of epilepsy are usually and perhaps correctly ascribed to the stigma of the label 'epileptic'. Nevertheless, patients' fears of death, brain damage and accidents due to epilepsy can play a significant role in the origins and maintenance of social isolation. Fear for their physical safety can keep many patients isolated, as they are afraid to go out of their homes because of possible seizures. The mythology surrounding 'being epileptic' produces many fears, including a dread of 'passing it on', mental deterioration and punishment from God.

Discussion topics

1. *Activities.*   Sports should be encouraged: the activity is selected according to each individual's particular seizure pattern.
2. *Alcohol.*   Warn about the dangers of drug and alcohol interactions.
3. *Denial.*   Discuss when denial is positive and when it is negative.
4. *Diagnosis.*   Explain how the diagnosis is reached and the significance of tests. Evaluate what the diagnosis means for each patient and family.
5. *Driving.*   Define the legal position at home and abroad.
6. *Employment.*   Consider interviews, attitudes and educating work colleagues. The emphasis should be on using the strengths of each person.
7. *Fits.*   Suggest simple precautions such as safety pillows, showers or shallow baths. Photosensitive people should sit 3 m from the television with a light on above the set.
8. *Heredity.*   The risk to a child born to a parent with epilepsy depends on the nature of the parent's epilepsy and the seizure threshold of both parents. Everyone has a seizure threshold level and is capable of having a fit in appropriate circumstances. A low threshold level can be passed on in a person's genetic structure.
9. *Insurance.*   Employers must be told that people are not high risks for accidents. Information about the British Epilepsy Association and its insurance scheme should be provided for newly diagnosed patients.
10. *Marriage.*   Fear of marriage and worries about sexual relations and fit frequency may have to be discussed. The nurse's aim is to help the person and his relatives to concentrate on a normal, full life.
11. *Pregnancy.*   Discuss medication and breast-feeding. When asked about terato-genic risks refer to current research findings that show that risk of damage to unborn babies is present but statistically very low.
12. *Prognosis.*   In most patients who develop seizures the epilepsy does not become chronic: early effective treatment may be important in order to prevent seizures from becoming intractable. One recent survey of a United Kingdom general practice found that the majority of patients suffered a small number of seizures only and that rapid and permanent remission was common once treatment had started. The condition becomes longstanding in about 20% of patients requiring medical

treatment. The prognosis for control of seizures was worse in those with partial or mixed seizures (Goodridge and Shorvon, 1983).

13. *Risks and precautions.* Discuss pillows, bathing, heights and other reasonable precautions. Trigger factors, such as television, stress, hunger, hyperventilation, over-tiredness, the premenstrual state, fever, alcohol and photic and other reflex stimuli, should be considered. Each individual has to identify his or her own triggers.

Dementing disorders

Dementia is defined as a global impairment of higher intellectual function in an alert patient (Harding, 1985). In a dementing condition the characteristic feature is a failure to grasp all the facets of a difficult situation; the person is said to be 'losing his grip'. As the disease progresses memory problems are more pronounced and the patient becomes completely disorientated, needing help with all the basic activities of living.

Patients who develop dementia because of some medically treatable condition, such as metabolic disease, vitamin deficiency, meningitis, a tumour or a vascular abnormality, will be dependent on the doctor to alleviate their problems. Patients who suffer from a dementing disorder for which there is no cure are most in need of nursing care; their relatives will rely on nurses and others to provide practical advice and support to help in the most demanding task of all, caring for a demented relative.

Alzheimer's disease

The most common type of illness involving dementia is senile dementia of the Alzheimer type (SDAT), or Alzheimer's disease as it is commonly known. The disease damages neurones and other brain tissue, interfering with the transmission of messages from cell to cell, and causing changes in behaviour. The onset is insidious: early symptoms include impaired memory for recent events with intact memory for remote events, decreased concern for others and a decreased ability to concentrate, to understand abstract concepts and to complete complex tasks. Depression with guilt and despondency are common in the early stages. As the disease progresses further aspects of dementia appear, such as outbursts of tears, spitefulness, aggression, a tendency to restlessness and disorientation from the surroundings. Impoverished language and difficulties in naming and word-finding are frequently present and the person is disorientated in time, place and person. Difficulty with feeding and dressing and a general deterioration of the person's personality will follow over a period of years. In the later stages speech sometimes undergoes a progressive disintegration so that the patient babbles incoherently and does not respond to command or verbal stimuli. Repetitive moaning or laughing are common. Gait disturbance and incontinence may appear, but generally quite late in the course of the illness. Finally the patient becomes bedridden and needs constant nursing. There are no specific treatments for Alzheimer's disease – at least, none that has been proved to be effective. Our greatest reliance is on drugs presumed to increase the metabolic activity in the injured brain, the so-called metabolic enhancers. The causes and the cure for Alzheimer's disease remain elusive.

Jakob–Creutzfeldt disease

Jakob–Creutzfeldt disease can generally be distinguished from other dementias by its relatively rapid course. This can be months rather than years from onset to death, but sometimes the course is prolonged. It is predominantly a disease of middle age, but some patients have been less than 30 years old. The disease is due to an unidentified slow virus infection.

Initially there is a sense of fatigue, apathy and some impairment of memory, accompanied by unpredictable behaviour. The second stage begins with signs of central nervous system involvement, epileptic convulsions, myoclonus, cortical blindness, akinetic mutism and characteristic EEG patterns. The patient is ataxic and the muscles of his arms and legs may atrophy. Spontaneous movements, tremor and dysarthria are almost invariably present.

Emotionally there may be a state of euphoria and incurable optimism alongside the obvious physical and mental disabilities. Anxiety and depression are also prominent clinical features. The patient has defective muscle control and subsequent spasticity of limbs. The actual disease phase lasts for a few months or 1–2 years, ending in a terminal phase of complete dementia with very severe manifestations of cerebral deficiency.

Huntington's chorea

Huntington's chorea is a progressive and incurable disease of the central nervous system transmitted through an autosomal gene. Each child of an affected person has a 50 per cent chance of inheriting the responsible gene, but carriers cannot be identified until there are clinical signs of the disease itself. By the time these appear, a carrier may well have had children: roughly two-thirds develop symptoms after the age of 29 years (Thomas, 1982). Dementia is common in Huntington's chorea, although the rate of progression of intellectual decline and the manifestations may differ between individual patients. Mental changes gradually develop, usually a few years after the onset of the involuntary movements.

In the earliest phases patients and families may report a loss of both recent and remote memory and a general disorientation of cognitive skills. Most patients become inert, apathetic and irritable. Delusions may occur and outbursts of excitement are not uncommon. Dementia is most feared by those at risk, and rightly so, because many consider this problem to be the most resistant to any type of therapeutic intervention.

Wilson's disease

Dementia in this disease may cause a general learning disability which takes the form of a rather sudden deterioration in the quality of schoolwork of adolescents, an inability to concentrate or read, memory loss or confusion about life and its activities (Scheinberg and Sternlieb, 1984). However, although Marsden (1987) says 'Cognitive changes undoubtedly occur in Wilson's disease, even to the extent of a frank dementia,' he observes that 'It is striking how many patients presenting with a severe movement disorder have relative preservation of intellect in the face of disastrous motor deficits.' The untreated patient with an advanced form of the disease is unable to express himself by speech or writing, drools copiously and, making only animal noises, may be thought to be mentally impaired. However, as Sternlieb et al (1987) explain: 'Most often there is imprisoned in this neurological catastrophe an individual with an intact intellect who is fully aware of his predicament and, consequently, angrily frustrated in the extreme.' One woman commented after her recovery that 'the most frustrating part of the whole experience is having intelligence and not being able to communicate – because people prejudge you as an idiot' (Scheinberg and Sternlieb, 1984).

Future hopes

The great interest in dementing diseases currently being shown by neuroscientists, pharmaceutical companies, research councils and families of the victims of these diseases should lead, in the not too distant future, to a better knowledge of and treatment for them.

Maintaining the demented person's residual skills, or even reducing the rate of decline, could improve the patient's quality of life. Many patients with dementia are affected by their environment. There have been a few reports of improved function following the introduction of stimulating activities and physical exercise in psycho-geriatric wards. Changes to the physical environment have also led to changes in behaviour. When efforts have been made to create natural social situations in the ward, or encourage the use of activity materials, social interaction and activity levels do increase (Woods, 1983). Ideally, the environment should be geared to the individual's skills, abilities and interests and should seek to maintain the skills the person does have.

Many demented patients are capable of learning. This learning ability is severely limited, but it does exist, and can be maximised using appropriate training techniques. Re-learning of verbal orientation has been extensively studied through an approach called *reality orientation* (RO). In RO the person is brought into contact with his surroundings and what is going on around him, both in informal contact with staff and in small group sessions of three to four patients and one or two staff, typically lasting 30 minutes and held several times each week. Research findings suggest that small changes in verbal orientation (e.g., knowing what day it is, the place, current events, etc.) usually result from RO programmes (Holden and Woods, 1982).

The majority of individuals who suffer from dementia live in the community, often supported by relatives. Arranging the environment to maintain skills and learning to use memory aids in the person's home are important and can be reinforced at day centres. Some relatives are able to incorporate these positive approaches into their own methods of coping with the demented person; others, perhaps, have coped by doing everything and feel too worn out to change.

Intracranial tumours

Tumour classification

The nurse needs sufficient information about intracranial tumours to be able to understand the different treatment procedures that each patient has and to communicate knowledgeably with patients and relatives. Unfortunately, the terminology involved is very elaborate, and not easily recalled, so this part of the chapter should be used mainly for reference purposes when the nurse learns that one of her patients has a cerebral tumour.

In the late 1970s an international panel convened by the World Health Organisation classified central nervous system tumours on the basis of their cells of origin and other histological features (Table 3.4).

Extrinsic (extra-axial) tumours

Most tumours are benign. Tumours grow slowly adjacent to the brain or the spinal cord and compress brain tissue without invading them. They can cause irreversible damage to adjacent normal tissue or cranial nerves. Examples:

- Meningioma
- Pituitary adenoma
- Craniopharyngioma
- Schwannoma (neuroma)
- Haemangioblastoma
- Metastatic tumour

Table 3.4   *Tumours*

Primary	Secondary
Extrinsic:	*Primary site*:
● Meninges – meningioma	● Female – breast
● Nerves – neurofibroma	● Male – prostate
● Glands – pituitary adenoma	● Both sexes – lung, alimentary tract, kidney, thyroid, skin
Intrinsic:	
● Glia – glioma	
● Ventricles – papilloma	
● Blood vessels – haemangioblastoma	
● Ependymal cells lining ventricles – ependymoma	
● Primitive cerebellar cells – medulloblastoma	

Intrinsic (intra-axial) tumours

Most tumours are malignant and grow within the substance of the nervous tissue. They develop more quickly than extrinsic tumours, infiltrating and destroying brain tissue as they spread. A few intrinsic tumours grow slowly (over 10–20 years) and so are viewed as relatively benign. Examples:

- Astrocytoma
- Oligodendroglioma
- Ependymoma
- Medulloblastoma

Primary tumours

Intracranial tumours may be *primary* if they arise from intracranial tissues, or *secondary* if they have spread from cancers elsewhere in the body. Primary tumours vary in their rate of growth, but rarely form metastatic deposits inside the skull: the majority are derived from glia, the meninges, the Schwann cells of the cranial nerves and the pituitary gland (Table 3.5). Gliomas are the most common primary brain tumours. Destruction of the cerebral cortex may cause weakness of the limbs, sensory impairment and, if in the dominant hemisphere, dysphasia. Focal symptoms may also be due to compression of isolated cranial nerves, and tumours in the cerebellum produce ataxia, dysarthria and nystagmus. Tumours may also cause focal or generalised epilepsy.

Secondary tumours

Tumours that originate in some extracranial organ such as a lung or breast are called secondary tumours. Such tumours consist of nodules surrounded by softened and oedematous brain tissue and are often multiple and scattered throughout the brain; they grow and disseminate rapidly. Metastatic tumours can be deposited anywhere inside or outside the brain and are, therefore, capable of producing any combination of symptoms. Other sources are the stomach and kidney. It has been estimated that 12 per

Table 3.5 *Incidence of intracranial tumours (Data from Snyder, 1983; Walton, 1977)*

Type of tumour	Percentages
Glioma	50
Meningioma	10–15
Pituitary adenoma	5–8
Acoustic neuroma	2–5
Metastatic	20
Others	5

cent of intracranial tumours are metastatic lesions from other cancerous sites. (See Chapter 5, 'Stephen'.)

Classification of malignancy

The criteria for the definition of malignancy in the central nervous system (CNS) tumours differ from those applied to other cancers. It is most unusual for primary CNS tumours to metastasise to other parts of the body. However, many have a tendency to invade locally and to recur after excision. Intracranial tumours are graded according to cellular composition and expected destructive changes such as thickening (hyperplasia), death (necrosis) and haemorrhage within tumour tissues. Even a tumour that is histologically benign and growing slowly may ultimately be lethal because of the space it occupies and the pressure it exerts on vital functions. There is, however, a classification based on clinical experience, with different tumours from Grade I (benign) to Grade IV (highly malignant). The clinical picture depends on both the rate of growth of the tumour and its site.

- Grade I – benign
- Grade II – semi-benign
- Grade III – relatively malignant
- Grade IV – highly malignant

Primary intrinsic tumours

Glioma

Gliomas are tumours derived from the cells that constitute the supporting tissue of the nervous system. A glioma develops from the glia; a meningioma from the meninges; ependymomas from the linings of the ventricles; neurofibromas from peripheral nerves and pituitary gland tumours from the pituitary gland. As gliomas are infiltrative tumours, which blend into normal surrounding brain without a well-defined border total excision is almost impossible.

Glioblastoma

These are highly malignant tumours of Grades II–IV. Cysts form in the tumour and their drainage is a great help to the patient's condition.

Astrocytoma

Astrocytomas can occur almost anywhere in the brain and vary in malignancy from Grade I–IV. A cystic astrocytoma can grow very slowly over many years but others grow exceedingly rapidly over a few weeks or months. The presenting signs and symptoms vary according to the site and size of the lesion. Cerebellar tumours that disturb the VIth and VIIth cranial nerves produce ataxia and uncoordinated movements. (See Chapter 5, 'Rebecca'.)

Oligodendrocytoma

This is a very slow-growing tumour of malignancy Grade I–IV. It often has calcium laid down in it, which can be seen on a straight X-ray of the skull.

Ependymoma

Primarily a slow growing tumour of childhood, an ependymoma is usually attached to the floor of the fourth ventricle and may infiltrate adjacent brain. It is of Grades I–IV.

Primary extrinsic tumour

Acoustic neurofibroma

This is a benign tumour that grows slowly, with little complaint from the patient. It is not malignant but may eventually not only compress the fibres of the VIIIth cranial nerve but also involve the facial, abducens and trigeminal nerves. The tumour develops in middle-aged people and produces deafness, facial paralysis and numbness. It also compresses the cerebellum resulting in ataxia, dysarthria and nystagmus. By obstructing the outflow of cerebrospinal fluid from the ventricles, it eventually gives rise to raised intracranial pressure.

An acoustic neurofibroma can be totally removed by microsurgical methods, but this may be difficult because it lies very close to the medulla and pons and to the centres concerned with cardiac and respiratory control in the brain-stem. The chance of removing the tumour safely as well as preserving the facial nerve is much higher if the tumour is small. (See Chapter 5, 'Sheila'.)

Meningioma

This is the second most common primary brain tumour. It is slow-growing, with signs and symptoms depending on where it is situated, and can grow to a huge size before producing any symptoms (headache and seizures) at all. A meningioma compresses the brain from outside and, being encapsulated, does not infiltrate the brain tissue; it can usually be completely removed surgically and only rarely recurs. Occasionally, complete removal may be impossible if the tumour lies close to a vital artery or venous sinus and cannot be separated from it without the risk of intractable haemorrhage.

Pituitary tumour

As the pituitary gland controls all the other hormone-producing glands, a tumour in this area may result in either too much or too little secretion of hormones. The most common tumour of the pituitary gland is, however, a chromophobe adenoma, which does not cause hormonal imbalance. It expands within the pituitary fossa (Figure 3.1), resulting in the destruction of the gland. A prolactinoma causes amenorrhoea or infertility in females and impotence in males. The symptoms of hypopituitarism

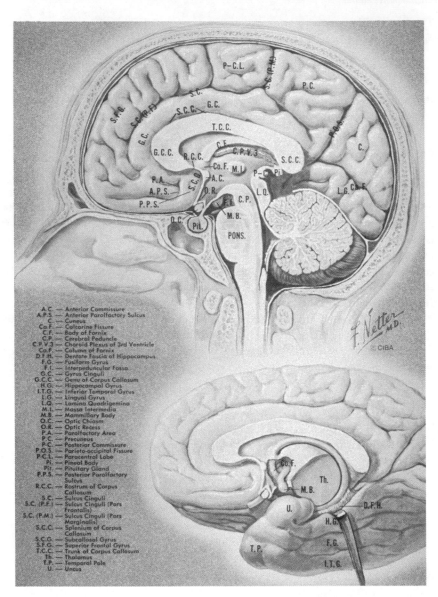

Figure 3.1 The pituitary gland (from *Ciba Collection of Medical Illustrations*, Vol. 1, p. 40. Reproduced by kind permission of Ciba-Geigy plc, Basle, all rights reserved)

develop insidiously and may be neglected for several years: reduction of body hair, increase in weight and intolerance of cold are commonly found. Expansion beyond the confines of the fossa compresses the optic chiasm, eventually giving rise to a bitemporal hemianopia. Ultimately, there is bilateral blindness, although the patient may initially be unaware of his diminishing visual fields and complains only of headache and blurring of central vision. After the tumour has been seen on a scan film and all other possible causes of the lesion have been excluded, surgical treatment will be planned to prevent further deterioration of vision. Most patients experience improvement within a few weeks postoperatively. (See Chapter 5, 'Susan'.)

Neurological deficits from tumours

Anosmia, visual deficits and, if the motor area is involved, hemiparesis.	
Distortion of sensory perceptions, agnosias, agraphia, receptive aphasia, focal seizures, dyspraxia, visual deficits, e.g. lower quadrantic hemianopia.	Parietal lobe
Visual defects, partial epilepsy with complex symptoms, flashing lights occurring just before the seizure.	Occipital lobe
Receptive dysphasia, upper quadrantic hemianopia, psychomotor and generalised seizures where olfactory or gustatory hallucinations predominate.	Temporal lobe
Loss of equilibrium in erect posture, ataxia.	Cerebellum
Deafness, tinnitus, unsteady gait, weakness, impairment of corneal reflex.	Cerebellopontine angle
Motor and sensory deficits, vomiting, deafness, dysphagia, dysfunction of cranial nerves IV–XII.	Brain-stem
Ataxia and uncoordinated movements, obstruction to flow of cerebrospinal fluid, dysfunction of cranial nerves VIII–XII.	Cerebellum

Spinal tumours

Spinal tumours occur at any age, although the commonest age is between 20 and 60, in both men and women. The tumours manifest themselves by pressure on the cord and nerve roots and by interfering with the blood supply. Spinal tumours can be classified according to their position in relation to the cord and covering membranes. Whereas most brain tumours are malignant, most spinal tumours are benign.

Intrinsic

Intrinsic tumours are most common in the cervical region. They first damage the sensory fibres that cross each other in the centre of the cord and produce a large patch of loss of sensation to pain and temperature over the arms and the upper part of the body. Later they spread to involve the motor fibres in the pyramidal tracts and cause paralysis of the legs. These tumours cannot be fully removed but their rate of growth is very slow. Secondary deposits grow in the spaces around the cord and develop very rapidly; attempts at removal or treatment by radiotherapy are rarely successful.

Extradural

These tumours are found in the spinal canal outside or above the dura in the extradural fat; they usually arise from the vertebrae or are secondary carcinomas spreading from the breast, prostate, lung or thyroid gland. They tend to destroy the vertebrae, causing collapse and consequent compression of the spinal cord and nerve roots (Schott, 1975).

Intradural extramedullary

These tumours are found inside the dura against the spinal cord. Commonly, these tumours are derived from the meninges (meningiomas) or the nerve roots (neurinomas or neurofibromas). They are benign, slow-growing and amenable to complete, permanent surgical removal.

Intramedullary

Five to ten per cent of malignant tumours arise in the spinal cord itself and are usually gliomas of varying degrees of malignancy. The commonest tumours are malignant lesions of the supporting cells (gliomas) and of the cells lining the central canal in the middle of the cord (ependymomas).

Symptoms

Intramedullary tumours typically have a very slowly progressive course, in some instances extending over 2 or 3 years, before definite physical findings appear. Very often the first symptoms are sensory: loss of sensation and unpleasant sensations of coldness are common and burning or constricting pain is felt in the distribution of the affected nerve roots. Bowel and bladder complaints occur earlier with intramedullary tumours than with those arising outside the cord. As the tumour grows the cord is displaced and then compressed.

Treatment

If diagnosis and treatment are delayed, the compression may result in irreversible damage to the cord (Draper, 1980). The surgical removal of benign extramedullary tumours is highly successful.

Prognosis

The prognosis will depend on the type of tumour and whether or not it can be removed. Extramedullary tumours are easier to excise than intramedullary ones. If intramedullary growths are operable, some damage to the cord and nerves is very possible. If the tumour can be successfully removed, recovery is often good, provided extensive destruction of cells and nerve fibres has not taken place, but it is usually slow and may take a year or more.

Myasthenic syndromes

Myasthenia gravis

The illness itself is not one homogeneous entity and can vary from involvement of the eye muscles alone to a severe generalised form. The mean age of onset is about 26 years in women and 30 years in men, but the condition may arise for the first time in childhood and occasionally as late as 80 years old. The onset is usually gradual and ptosis of one or both upper lids is often the first symptom, soon to be associated with diplopia due to paralysis of one or more of the external ocular muscles.

In the mildest form of myasthenia only the ocular muscles are affected: this gives rise to ptosis and/or diplopia, often with some restriction of lateral and upward gaze. If the myasthenia remains confined to the extraocular muscles for over a year the symptoms rarely become generalised. The most active stage of the disease is during its first 5 years, during which time there may be a threat to life; thereafter, the risk to life is less, but there may be serious continuing disability. The course of the disease may be punctuated by temporary improvement and worsening. Spontaneous remissions occur in a quarter of patients but these rarely last for more than 2 years and are not usually repeated.

Deterioration in the patient's condition may sometimes be related to undue physical activity, infection, childbirth or emotional disturbance, when the muscle weakness may become worse and spread to previously unaffected muscles. In severe cases the weakness of the upper limbs is such that the hands cannot be lifted to the mouth and it is characteristic that although muscle power may initially be reasonably satisfactory, the strength rapidly declines after testing a particular movement on several occasions. Pharyngeal and respiratory muscle weakness are the major life-threatening symptoms of myasthenia gravis. After the disease has been in progress for 10 years death from myasthenia itself is rare and in some instances the disease is apparently burnt out by this stage (Walton 1977; Scadding and Havard, 1981). (See Chapter 5, 'Patricia' and 'Rosemary'.)

Eaton–Lambert syndrome

In this syndrome, muscular fatiguability with weakness and wasting affects the proximal parts of the limbs and trunk; occasionally the external ocular and bulbar muscles are also involved. The weakness is often myasthenic in the sense that the patient complains of fatigue after exertion but it has been observed that muscle power may in fact increase after brief exercise, a reversed myasthenic effect. There is a failure of acetylcholine release at the neuromuscular junction. The syndrome may be distinguished from true myasthenia gravis by electromyography. This syndrome is generally associated with oat cell carcinoma of the bronchus (Draper, 1980).

Myasthenic and cholinergic crisis

Both myasthenic and cholinergic crisis produce acute respiratory failure. Myasthenic crisis is due to inadequate anticholinesterase medication, while cholinergic crisis results from too much. Medical management of either of these conditions includes correction of respiratory failure as the first priority; this correction may require intubation, tracheostomy or assisted ventilation.

In myasthenic crisis an intravenous injection of 2 mg Tensilon (edrophonium chloride) will improve weakness. An increase in anticholinesterase drugs is then necessary and the patient may require respirator care. If sweating, vomiting or pallor occur, a cholinergic crisis may be starting; the patient may then require assisted respiration and intravenous atropine injections at about hourly intervals (Ashworth and Saunders, 1985).

Physiology

The weakness of muscles that rapidly worsens as the muscle is used and recovers with rest occurs in patients with myasthenia gravis because of abnormal neuromuscular activity. Myasthenia gravis is an autoimmune disease, with circulating antibodies that attack the enzyme receptors in the neuromuscular junctions (Figure 3.2), preventing impulses from passing from the motor nerves to the muscle fibres. Acetylcholinergic drugs are used for treating patients medically because this is the chemical involved at the neuromuscular junction to stimulate muscle responses to nervous stimuli.

The thymus gland is abnormal in 75 per cent of patients with myasthenia, often being markedly enlarged. Up to 15 per cent of patients have a thymoma, which is a malignant tumour of the gland, usually encapsulated and slow-growing (Wilson, 1979).

Treatment

The approach to treatment can take one of three routes: pharmacological, immunological or surgical, i.e. thymectomy. The pharmacological approach uses anticholinesterase drugs such as pyridostigmine (Mestinon) and neostigmine (Prostigmin), which improve

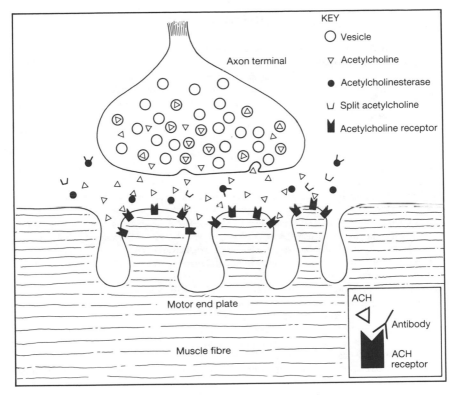

Figure 3.2 Motor neurone junction

neuromuscular transmission by prolonging the action of acetylcholine by inhibiting the enzyme anticholinesterase. Such treatment can sometimes be fully effective in very mildly affected patients and useful as supplementary treatment in severe forms of the condition.

Patients who have ocular or milder myasthenia are given alternate-day predniso-lone corticosteroid therapy, with a gradually decreasing dose until the minimum has been found that will control their symptoms. The need for long-term maintenance treatment for most patients has to be accepted, providing an 80 per cent remission rate. In more severely affected patients alternate-day corticosteroid therapy supplemented by plasma exchange on four or five daily exchanges may be the most effective therapy. When symptoms are adequately controlled immunosuppressive drugs are slowly reduced with the aim of defining the minimum maintenance dose.

If symptoms are generalised and more than minimal, thymectomy is indicated in those whose illness began under the age of about 45–50 years. If a thymoma is present, it has to be removed as it presses on the mediastinum.

References

Ashworth B and Saunders M (1985) *Management of Neurological Disorders*. London: Butterworths.

Bickerstaff E R (1987) *Neurology*, 4th edn. London: Hodder and Stoughton.

Chadwick D and Usiskin S (1987) *Living with Epilepsy*. London: Macdonald Optima.

Draper I T (1980) *Lecture Notes on Neurology*, 5th edn. Oxford: Blackwell Scientific.

Goodridge D M G and Shorvon S D (1983) Epileptic seizures in a population of 6000. *British Medical Journal*, **287**: 641–647.

Harding A E (1985) Degenerative disorders. In: *Neurology*, Ross Russell R and Wiles C M (eds.), pp. 187–203. London: William Heinemann

Hayden M R (1981) *Huntington's Chorea*. Berlin: Springer-Verlag.

Holden U and Woods B (1982) *Reality Orientation – Psychological Approaches to the 'Confused' Elderly*. Edinburgh: Churchill Livingstone.

Lawden M (1986) Gilles de la Tourette syndrome: a review. *Journal of the Royal Society of Medicine*, **79**: 282–288.

Lees A J, Robertson M, Trimble M R and Murray N M F (1984) A clinical study of Gilles de la Tourette syndrome in the United Kingdom. *Journal of Neurology, Neurosurgery and Psychiatry*, **47**: 1–8.

Lees A J (1985) *Tics and Related Disorders*. Edinburgh: Churchill Livingstone.

Lishman W A (1987) *Organic Psychiatry: The Psychological Consequences of Cerebral Disorder*, 2nd edn. Oxford: Blackwell Scientific.

Marsden C D (1987) Wilson's disease. *Quarterly Journal of Medicine*, New Series, **65** (248): 959–966.

Newrick P G and Langton-Hewer R (1984) Motor neurone disease; can we do better? A study of 42 patients. *British Medical Journal*, **289**(2): 539–542.

Newsom-Davis J (1982) Myasthenia. In: *Advanced Medicine 18*, Sarner M (ed.), pp. 149–159. London: Pitman.

Norris F H, Smith R A and Denys E H (1985) Motor neurone disease: towards better care. *British Medical Journal*, **291**(2): 259–262.

Rose A S (1979) Long-term care of patients with multiple sclerosis: a neurologist's perspective. *Neurology*, **30**(2): 59–61.

Russell R W S (1983) Symptomatology of optic neuritis. *Bulletin of the Society of Belgian Ophthalmology*, **208**(1): 127–130.

Scadding G F and Havard C W H (1981) Pathogenesis and treatment of myasthenia gravis. *British Medical Journal*, **283**(2): 1008–1012.

Scheinberg I H and Sternlieb I (1984) *Wilson's Disease*. Philadelphia: W B Saunders.

Schott G D (1975) Spinal tumours 1. Classification. *Nursing Times*, **71**(52): 2055–2057.

Snyder M (1983) Appendix: brain tumours. In: *Guide to Neurological and Neurosurgical Nursing*, Snyder M (ed.), p. 580. New York: John Wiley and Sons.

Stell R, Thompson P D and Marsden C D (1988) Botulinum toxin in spasmodic torticollis. *Journal of Neurology, Neurosurgery and Psychiatry*, **51**(7): 920–923.

Sternlieb I, Giblin D R and Scheinberg H (1987) Wilson's disease. In: *Movement Disorders II*, Marsden C D and Fahn S (eds.), pp. 288–302. London: Butterworths.

Stevens D L (1982) *Huntington's Chorea: A Booklet for Family Doctors and Other Professionals*. Leicestershire: Association to Combat Huntington's Chorea.

Thomas S (1982) Ethics of a predictive test for Huntington's chorea. *British Medical Journal*, **284**(1): 1383–1385.

Tibbets R W (1981) Neuropsychiatric aspects of tics and spasms. *British Journal of Hospital Medicine*, **25**(5): 454–464.

Trimble M R (1983) The Gilles de la Tourette syndrome. *Psychiatry in Practice*, **2**(17): 7–14.

Walton J N (1977) *Brain's Diseases of the Nervous System*, 8th edn. Oxford: Oxford University Press.

Wilson S (1979) A cure is in sight. *Nursing Mirror*, **148**(1): 17–20.

Woods B (1983) Senile dementia – positive psychological approaches. *Bethlem & Maudsley Gazette*, **31**(1): 8–9.

Further reading

Cerebrovascular disease

Ancowitz A (1975) *Strokes and Their Prevention: How To Avoid High Blood Pressure and Hardening of the Arteries.* New York: Van Nostrand Reinhold.

Clark M (1983) Diary of a stroke victim. *Nursing Times,* **79**(34): 27–30.

Francis M (1983) Shipwrecked in my body. *Nursing Mirror,* **156**(25): 45–47.

Mackay A and Nias B C (1979) Strokes in the young and middle-aged: consequences to the family and to society. *Journal of the Royal College of Physicians of London,* **13**(2): 106–112.

Mackintosh A (1984) *The Heart Disease Reference Book: Direct and Clear Answers to Everyone's Questions.* London: Harper and Row.

Macphee M (1984) Like being hit by a hammer. *Nursing Mirror,* **158**(22): 31–33.

Myco F (1983) *Nursing Care of the Hemiplegic Stroke Patient.* London: Harper and Row.

Pulhopek M (1980) Stroke: an update on vascular disease. *Journal of Neurosurgical Nursing,* **12**(2): 81–87.

Sears E and Poulson S (1983) Intracranial haemorrhage. *Nursing,* **2**(15): 436–440.

Yeung Laiwah A C (1982) Transient cerebral ischaemic attacks. *Journal of the Royal College of Physicians,* **16**(2): 117–122.

Degenerative disorders

Cochrane G M (1987) *Management of Motor Neurone Disease.* London: MNDA/Churchill Livingstone.

Forsythe E (1988) *Multiple Sclerosis: Exploring Sickness and Health.* London: Faber and Faber.

Maclellan M (1989) Community care of a patient with multiple sclerosis. *Nursing,* **3**(33): 28–32.

Matthews B (1985) *Multiple Sclerosis: The Facts,* 2nd edn. Oxford: Oxford University Press.

Small O (1986) Huntington's chorea. *Nursing Times,* **82**(15): 32–33.

Movement disorders

Duvoisin R C (1984) *Parkinson's Disease: A Guide for Patient and Family,* 2nd edn. New York: Raven Press.

Essex L (1983) One patient's view of Parkinson's Disease. *Journal of Royal Society of Health,* **103**(5): 169–173.

Gresh C (1980) Helpful tips for patients with Parkinson's Disease. *Nursing (USA),* **10**(1): 26–33.

Holt P (1983) Parkinson's Disease. *Nursing (UK),* **2**(15): 448–450.

Manson L and Caird F I (1985) Survey of hobbies and transport of patients with Parkinson's Disease. *British Journal of Occupational Therapy,* **48**(7): 199–200.

Stern G and Lees A (1982) *Parkinson's Disease: The Facts.* Oxford: Oxford University Press.

The epilepsies

Chadwick D and Usiskin S (1987) *Living with Epilepsy.* London: Macdonald Optima.

Jeavons P M and Aspinall A (1985) *The Epilepsy Reference Book.* London: Harper and Row.

Laidlaw J, Richens A and Oxley J (eds.) (1988) *A Textbook of Epilepsy,* 3rd edn. Edinburgh: Churchill Livingstone.

Laidlaw M V and Laidlaw J (1984) *People with Epilepsy.* Edinburgh: Churchill Livingstone.

McGovern S (1982) *The Epilepsy Handbook.* London: Sheldon Press.

Reynolds E H and Trimble M R (1981) *Epilepsy and Psychiatry.* Edinburgh: Churchill Livingstone.

Dementing disorders

Sandeman P O, Norberg A, Adolfson R, Axelsson K and Hedly V (1986) Morning care of patients with Alzheimer-type dementia: a theoretical model based on direct observations. *Journal of Advanced Nursing,* **11**(4): 369–378.

Stewart-Dedman M (1988) Strain and strategy. *Nursing Times*, **84**(17): 38–41.
Wertheimer J and Marois M (eds.) (1984) *Senile Dementia: Outlook for the Future*. New York: Liss.
Zarit S H, Orr N K and Zarit J M (1985) *The Hidden Victims of Alzheimer's Disease: Families Under Stress*. New York: New York University Press.

Intracranial tumours

Macrae A (1984) Cerebral tumours. *Nursing Mirror*, **158**(17): 36–38.
Tortorelli B A (1981) Acoustic neuroma: an overview of the disorder and nursing care for these patients. *Journal of Neurosurgical Nursing*, **13**(4): 170–177.

Chapter 4

PSYCHOSOCIAL ASPECTS OF NEUROLOGICAL DISORDER

Chapter theme

There can be little doubt that nursing is a stressful occupation that requires a uniformity of spirit and conformity of action for its survival. Traditionally, the 'good' nurse is speedy, efficient, non-communicative and non-responsive to cues from patients, whether verbal or otherwise. To overlook a person's feelings about his illness may not only retard the healing process but may actually prevent it. To overcome the depersonalising effect of hospital specialisation the nurse in daily contact with patients should get to know the person behind the diagnostic label.

Some nurses and doctors who join the management team seem, almost overnight, to forget their earlier concerns about patients and professional colleagues. In those institutions where senior nurses fail to support clinically based staff one hears comments such as, 'No one is interested in what we think, we only look after the patients'. Work appraisal for the nurse may be limited to a threatening interview only when her performance is unsatisfactory: this is a major source of stress.

The nurse's role is to provide a simple, dignified and uncomplicated response to the patient, who expects kindness, understanding and emotional support when he approaches her for information. The patient needs a clear picture of his condition and what he can expect to happen, because such realistic basic knowledge helps him to structure his activities to feel part of a team and continue to feel responsible for his own life. Nursing is about knowing how to make someone else comfortable, instilling in another person that sense of being 'on top of it', even in a threatening situation, and encouraging a sense of endurance.

By contemplating the ideas presented in this chapter and by examining the attitudes and feelings of nurses and patients, a nurse can develop, in discussion with colleagues, a supportive system to improve and confirm her ability as a nurse. She must be comfortable with her own feelings and attitudes before she can develop constructive nurse–patient relationships.

Contents

Feelings

Most chronic illnesses show an individual physical deterioration over time. This may be a rapid process or characterised by plateaux where no physical changes occur for long periods. In contrast, patients who have had a cerebrovascular accident or head injury begin with a clear onset and are then at their most vulnerable. This tends to be followed, in the survivors, by a steady improvement. The most rapid improvements tend to occur in the first 3 months when patients may move from a comatose state to one where they may be mobile and able to converse with others. This rapid rate of recovery in the early stages frequently establishes expectations in the family that the patient will be left with no residual deficits. When the recovery slows down and where residual deficits remain, the family have difficulty in adjusting their expectations. The most difficult period occurs when the realisation takes place that the patient has reached a plateau and may not fully recover.

Psychological stamina refers to a unique resilience present in human beings. Despite the crisis of illness and day-to-day uncertainty, some patients are able to maintain a psychological equilibrium. Somehow events that could be viewed as threats are interpreted as being meaningful. At the other extreme, chronic illness may cause psychological imbalance. Depression and anxiety are two prevalent symptoms in individuals who are chronically ill. The extent to which a person 'goes to pieces' when he has to live with a chronically disabling neurological disorder depends upon his existing personality, the nature and extent of the disorder, where he is in the life-span and the support system surrounding him. Although some conditions are carried forward from childhood so that the individual has had time to adjust, he could as easily have learnt to become dependent and helpless. Other conditions occur suddenly, just when the person is about to develop his career or start a family. Alternatively, the onset is insidious, at the point when the individual faces maximum responsibilities in middle age. The disability in some conditions is periodical, while in others it is a progressive process. Some conditions provoke sympathy, others, like hearing and speech disorders, often provoke irritation and frustration. Many conditions are stigmatising, time-consuming or demand strict regimes.

Stroke (CVA)

Depression following a stroke has been found to occur in many patients, ranging from 26 to 45 per cent of selected patients studied (Newman, 1984). Robinson and Price (1982), in a survey of 103 patients attending a stroke clinic, found that one-third were depressed, the majority remaining so for at least 6 months. The peak incidence of depression was in the period 6 months to 2 years after the stroke had occurred.

Psychological problems can be severe when the life situation is profoundly altered as a consequence of the stroke. Many important sources of gratification, pleasure and interest may be lost both for the patient and for other family members. There are often far-reaching domestic upheavals, particularly in younger patients – the wife may need to work and the husband adjust to a new domestic role. Marital problems may come to the fore, with rejection or even desertion by the spouse (Lishman, 1987).

A person with communication and mobility difficulties cannot be as independent as he would like to be, and the increased reliance on others may exacerbate any existing conflicts over dependency. Considerable frustration is experienced by someone who wishes to communicate but is unable to do so; he feels imprisoned by his frustration and this may lead to a negative attitude to life. A patient with bowel and bladder incontinence struggles with issues related to control and autonomy; hemiplegic patients have changes in body image that lower frustration tolerance and raise anxiety levels.

The person who has had a cerebrovascular accident tends to tire easily when reading, talking or doing mental work; his powers of concentration may be impaired so that mental tasks may become more demanding and people begin to notice that he has memory problems. Fear and anxiety can be crippling psychologically: the patient fears further strokes, he is worried that he may fall, he fears being permanently crippled and he may be anxious about money problems. Angry outbursts are often directed towards the person who cares for the patient and this can be a common cause of domestic tension and resentment.

Excessive or inappropriate weeping or laughter can occur after a cerebrovascular accident. A few unfortunate patients laugh or cry when any attempt is made to converse with them. Some are provoked by conversation, especially with close relatives or when discussing discharge from hospital or some emotional subject; others may only be provoked by a specific enquiry about the symptom itself. These may be outbursts in which frustration, anger and depression are combined as, for example, with the patient who, when asked to do something he could previously perform with ease, now finds that he cannot and is unable to inhibit his emotions and breaks into sobbing, expressing his sense of hopelessness.

In the longer term the stresses and adjustments caused by a cerebrovascular accident in the family may result in some emotional disturbance, in particular depression, in other family members. Coughlan and Humphrey (1982) showed that 25 per cent of spouses received treatment for depression or tension in a 3–8-year follow-up period: this group had not received treatment for these disorders before their spouse's illness.

Changed body image

Body image is the ability to feel a limb, to appreciate the movements of the joints and to appreciate a limb's place in space and its relationship to the body. Body image is built up by the sense of muscular position, known as *proprioception*: this sense is dependent on impulses from muscles, joints and tendons by which the body knows itself, and judges with perfect, automatic, instantaneous precision the position and motion of all its movable parts, their relation to one another and their alignment in space.

Disorders of body image relate to a poor sense of the position of one's body in space, which may be unilateral, affecting only one side of the body (that opposite to the side of brain damage), or bilateral. Impairments in body awareness lead to great difficulties for the patient in the activities of daily living. He may neglect one side of his body when washing, dressing or shaving. By steadily and repeatedly encouraging the patient to attend to his neglected side, the nurse may reduce the extent of the neglect.

Our mental awareness of our body's size and its relationship to other objects can be disturbed by brain lesions, such as a stroke, which affects certain areas of the brain. A patient may complain that one side of his body, or a limb, is not there or feels as if it does not belong to him, or that half his body may feel abnormally large or small. Such episodes may be short and caused by transient ischaemic attacks, migraine or epilepsy. In a longer-lasting condition the patient may not use one side of his body fully and, in the severe form, may actually deny that half of his body exists. In another form of distortion of body image a patient with paralysed limbs may deny that he is paralysed and be convinced that he moves when asked to do so.

The changes in sensation following a stroke depend upon which side of the brain has been damaged. Touch (tactile) sensation seems more widely represented in the right hemisphere. This means that a right-hand sensory impairment tends to occur only after damage to the sensorimotor area of the left hemisphere, whereas a deficit in the left hand can be caused by damage in one of a number of areas in the right hemisphere. Sensory impairments tend to show recovery during rehabilitation.

Salter (1988) explains that

> the patient with a slowly progressive change in body image, such as the often gradual weakening experienced in multiple sclerosis, may be able to cope more effectively with that change than someone involved in traumatic paraplegia. The person with multiple sclerosis may progress from walking stick to a frame, then to a wheelchair; he may well feel frustrated and angry as each step on the downward slope means more loss of independence.

Patients who have suffered from rigidity for some years often feel very disorientated and lacking in confidence when they have to re-learn 'normal' balance reactions and re-educate the body image for functional activities (Downie, 1986).

Patients' reactions

Patients vary in their reaction to any kind of disability and disfigurement. Some may appear very distressed while others seem to cope quickly and with few problems. How the patient copes will depend upon his own attitudes and values and his own body image: if it is changed and fails to match up to what he previously felt was normal and acceptable both to himself and others, the effect can be very disturbing. He may feel ashamed, inferior or angry and, depending on how visible the change is, these feelings can be reinforced by others whom he meets. Sometimes after the change in body image the loss of self-esteem may be so great that the patient fears social contact and takes steps to avoid it.

Some stoics believe that they must bear bravely what God has allowed them to suffer and feel that they will be rewarded in the after life; others feel only shame with their affliction and may be treated as outcasts by their families or religious leaders (Salter, 1988).

A man who always put great value on taking his wife and children to various destinations by car, and regarded himself as an important manager of the household, may at first be devastated when he has to lose his driving licence because of epilepsy. He will need to rethink his whole outlook on life, come to terms with new limitations and set himself different goals. The new state may make him feel ashamed or inferior. He will need reassurance that he is no less a person just because of, for example, an epileptic disorder.

A patient's experience

Sacks (1987) encountered a bull on a desolate mountain in Norway, which left him with a severely damaged leg. He describes his disturbed body image:

> I knew not my leg. It was utterly strange, not mine, unfamiliar. I gazed upon it with absolute non-recognition. The more I gazed at that cylinder of chalk, the more alien and incomprehensible it appeared to me. I could no longer feel it as 'mine,' or as part of me. It seemed to bear no relation whatever to me. It was absolutely not me – and yet, impossibly, it was attached to me – and even more impossibly, 'continuous' with me . . . When I closed my eyes, I had no feeling whatever of where the leg lay – no feeling that it was 'here', as opposed to 'there', no feeling that it was anywhere – no feeling at all.

The nurse's role

> Whether a nurse works on a particular ward or unit, in the out-patient department, or is a community or specialist nurse, one of her primary functions is to help patients as they try to come to terms with their lot in life, and if that includes a change in the way that they see themselves, it is inevitable that she will want to help . . . help them to see themselves as whole human beings . . . Through a nurse's work with patients, although she may have to leave them with their physical imperfections, she is able to relieve them of permanent emotional scars. Remember, too, that not all fruits ripen at the same time (Salter, 1988).

Parkinson's disease

'Melancholy' was a term used by James Parkinson to describe the 'unhappy sufferer' or patients with the 'shaking palsy'. Frequently, a carer will express sadness and disappointment that, just at the time when the couple had looked forward to or had entered retirement for which they had made plans, Parkinson's disease had turned her companion into a dependant.

Most detailed descriptions of the clinical manifestations of this disease have included depression, the cause of which is unknown (Nanton, 1985). The depression is often described as reactive in nature, setting in immediately the patient is informed of the nature of the disease or developing later as an understandable response to disablement. In addition, however, some authors say that depression is part of the disease process itself, but Lishman (1987) and Nanton (1985) identified several investigations that failed to show a relationship between the severity of depression and the degree of disability resulting from Parkinson's disease. Quite often, the depression responded to antidepressive treatment (including electroconvulsive therapy) while the disability persisted unchanged.

Multiple sclerosis

Since it was first described over 150 years ago, multiple sclerosis has been identified with a variety of emotional disturbances, including depression, euphoria and hysteria. The degree of depression in multiple sclerosis can be severe and suicide has been reported in a considerable number of cases. Attention has also been directed to the possibility that psychological factors may be important in precipitating fresh relapses of the disease (Lishman, 1987).

Depression is the most logical and understandable response to the patient's predicament in the earlier stages, whereas euphoria is more typical as the disease progresses. The transition over a period of time from depression to euphoria can sometimes be clearly observed in the individual patient. Whether or not the patient experiences depression depends on the psychological impact of his disability. Sphincter disturbances are an especially severe psychological trauma, increasing dependency and often meaning the end of sexual relationships.

Examination of the relationship between age, severity of physical disability and duration of illness does not enable one to predict whether or not a person will experience psychological problems in the future. There is, however, agreement that patients with multiple sclerosis do not comprise a uniform group of individuals with the same problems.

Dementia – personality

An attitude frequently noticed in the person who is dementing is one of denial that he has an illness problem. When this is added to the inability to concentrate, persuading the person that he really does need to visit a doctor is very difficult. Mental confusion can change a person's personality so that she or he is barely recognisable as 'Mum' or 'Dad', or may not even recognise the carer. This distressing behaviour can put a great strain on family relationships.

> Once firmly established the disintegration of intellect and personality proceeds relentlessly. Episodes of confusion and delirium may occur at night and the patient sleeps badly. Repetitive futile behaviour is characteristic and restlessness may become extreme. Psychotic features are common, usually of a paranoid nature and sometimes with grotesque hypochondriacal delusions. Emotions become blunted, though outbursts of anger may occur if routines are disturbed. Habits deteriorate with loss of sphincter control, so that the patient is sometimes found to have been living in appalling conditions by the time he is admitted to hospital. The appearance becomes decrepit and shrunken, and the gait slow, shuffling and tottery (Lishman, 1987).

Movement disorders

Wilson's disease

A literature survey by Scheinberg and Sternlieb (1984) revealed that:

> Almost every patient with Wilson's disease suffers at some time during the course of his disease from a psychoneurosis, a manic-depressive or schizophrenic psychosis, or a disorder impossible to distinguish from these; bizarre behavioural abnormalities, often characterised by impulsivity and occasionally extending to criminal behaviour or a combination of any of the foregoing.

Much of the emotional disorder is probably the result of the patient's reaction to his disability, including tremor, rigidity, dystonia, dysarthria and dysphagia. However, personality change and other psychiatric disturbances have also been attributed to the widespread brain damage, apparent on the CT scan (Lishman, 1987).

Scheinberg and Sternlieb provide the following fascinating case studies:

> An 18-year-old man was hospitalized in a psychiatric institution for hostility, impulsivity and grandiose ideas. He asked his parents to bring him his clarinet so that, like a Pied Piper, he could lead all the patients off the ward. Despite the appearance of slurred speech, micrographia and tremors, noted by a number of physicians at age 20, psychotherapy alone was continued for another three years, by which time his neurological Wilson's disease was irreversible. Vigorous decoppering therapy had no appreciable benefit, and his disease progressed to total incapacity, anarthria and death.

> A 24-year-old man suffered from persistent compulsive voyeurism that began after he glimpsed the naked wife of a fellow air force officer. Following arrest, prison and a suicide attempt, psychotherapy was initiated. Tremors and uncoordination, first noted at age 27, progressed. Not until he was 30 did a doctor suspect Wilson's disease. Decoppering therapy and less frequent psychotherapy were followed by complete remission of all neurological and psychiatric signs and symptoms. Taking penicillamine alone for the last 20 years, he is married, the father of three children and the president of a prosperous business.

Gilles de la Tourette syndrome

In some people with the Gilles de la Tourette syndrome the severity of obsessive compulsive symptoms is the most obvious and disabling aspects of the disorder. These problems have been vividly described in one study (Frankel et al, 1986) where one patient indicated that it was hard to concentrate because of unwanted thoughts or images that came into his mind and would not go away; another person felt that some of the thoughts and feelings that occupied him were a senseless waste of time and energy.

Motor neurone disease

Motor neurone disease is an illness of losses: there is constant loss for the patient, carer and professionals. The carer feels frustration and sadness: 'Oh dear, now they can't do that'. The loss of independence, pride and self-sufficiency makes the sufferer feel worthless, as what he can do is diminishing with time.

At a Motor Neurone Disease (MND) Association multidisciplinary conference held in October 1988 Dame Cicely Saunders commented that 'Although 200 people with motor neurone disease have been through St Christopher's Hospice, every single one has been different.' The highlight of the day was when Mr and Mrs Smith described how they coped with the disease.

Ann Smith explained that although she was diagnosed in 1983, for many months before that she had had cramps, falls, and difficulty getting up and it took her longer to walk even a short distance. She then noticed flickering or twitching in the muscles of her legs (i.e. fasciculation). After many blood tests and an electromyelogram (EMG), she was then told the diagnosis and subsequent hospital visits relieved the sense of isolation, as 'Patients feel very lonely if they are never seen.' Reactions to the diagnosis were shock, fear and resentment. The patient and her husband needed to know as much as possible. Their consultant gave them time to ask questions and helped them to plan a new way of life.

As motor neurone disease sometimes progresses very fast, plans had to be made for the future. They contemplated moving to a bungalow but chose instead to renovate their existing house. The council tried to persuade them to move the bedroom to the ground floor, but they did not want the house to be dominated by disability, as they wished to live as normal a life as possible. They installed a lift from the ground floor to the bedroom upstairs, an extra downstairs toilet, enlarged the bathroom and strengthened the roof. An occupational therapist advised joining the MND Association.

Although Ann could go shopping and visit friends, she needed a few hours' sleep in the afternoon. A battery pavement car enabled her to retain some of her independence. There was a slow but steady deterioration; she found it a great help getting involved in the MND Association: 'they got strength from each other'. The most important thing was for she and her husband to spend as much time together as possible, so Mr Smith retired 6 years prematurely. By this time, Ann found she was having spasms in all parts of her body, as well as general muscle weakness, so that they had to get many aids, some of which they bought, others which were obtained from the Social Services. When Mr Smith had to go away for 2 weeks, Ann stayed in a hospice, which enabled her husband to have a break confident that she was being well cared for. Five years after the onset of the disease, Ann finds that her days are short because of extreme tiredness: the time she spent talking to conference participants would be followed by a day in bed to regain her strength.

Conference participants were encouraged to look at the loss experienced by families with motor neurone disease and share the sadness, setting realistic goals. As motor neurone disease is a terminal illness, the patients will eventually die. Sufferers have a long period of dealing with status, role change and identity. The nurse should be prepared to respond to a patient who asks, 'Do I matter?' or says, 'I feel very angry and can't speak.' Loss, grief, tears and anger should be accepted as necessary outlets of the frustrations of the disease. Keeping in touch with the bereaved relative may mean considering the most difficult part of the illness and how things could have been done differently. With good multidisciplinary teamwork, much can be achieved and regular family meetings can support both the family and the team.

Huntington's chorea

Every individual who has a close relative with Huntington's chorea is continually on the alert for any suspicious signs of the disorder and tries to master the disease through activity in the same way that people who very much fear going 'crazy' often pretend to be 'crazy'. Those people who have watched an affected parent change and decline from a familiar, healthy person to an unrecognisable stranger with bizarre movements, uncontrollable behaviour and slurred speech, probably did so during childhood, which often left them with a distorted understanding of the effects of the disease.

Wexler (1979) found that the primary concerns of vulnerable individuals were the intellectual deterioration and personality changes wrought by the disease, the socially embarrassing choreiform movements, regressive problems such as incontinence and, especially, the extreme dependence involved in becoming chronically ill. 'You can live with jerkiness but you can't live without your mind.' Nearly all had talked of 'becoming a vegetable', 'stagnating', 'going crazy', of not being able to communicate and of the terror of ending their lives in a mental institution. One of the most frequently voiced fears was of choking to death or dying of starvation.

Accompanying the physical symptoms are psychological signs ranging from boredom and depression to aggression, the latter usually being directed against close family members. Sometimes, there are definite psychiatric symptoms as well as dementia. With rare exceptions, all patients with Huntington's chorea have some type of personality change which has no particular pattern or sequence: anxiety, irritability, promiscuity and alcoholism have all been mentioned.

A striking feature of patients who have Huntington's chorea is their lack of concern about the illness, but this disinterest may also affect their work and social activities. Apathy may occur at all stages of the illness but it tends to be associated with the onset of intellectual decline as the dementia progresses. Schizophrenia-like symptoms such as persecutory delusions are not unusual in Huntington's chorea and may occur at any time during the illness, either with depression or alone. (See also Chapter 3, 'Degenerative disorders'.)

Attitudes

Loss

Impairment is characterised by a permanent or transitory psychological, physiological or anatomical loss or abnormality. It includes such defects as a missing or defective limb, organ, tissue or other structure of the body, or an abnormality of a functional system or mechanism of the body, including mental function. It thus represents any disturbance or interference with the normal structure and functioning of the body and the person. The existence of impairment may not necessarily be handicapping: a person who has lost both legs may well have a very hectic social life, whereas someone else with a minor facial blemish may never go out because of it.

Practicalities

A disability is any restriction or lack of the ability to perform an activity in the manner or within the range considered normal for a human being. This refers to the inability, or at least restricted ability, to perform normal personal or social tasks such as washing, dressing and household chores. External factors are also important: someone in a wheelchair in a non-adapted house may be limited functionally, but might not be in an adapted house. The less he is able to do, the more help he needs; the more help he needs, the more severely disabled he is. The extent to which a person is physically dependent on others represents the severity of his disability.

Citizenship

To some disabled people 'disability is something imposed on top of our impairments by the way we are unnecessarily isolated and excluded from full participation in society' (Campbell-Hayes, 1988). Any discussion about disablement is limited to consideration of the physical state of a small minority of people. Society is made up of the short and the tall, the dim and the bright, the calm and the volatile, the able-bodied and the disabled. If there exists somewhere a person whose body is in immaculate working order then he is the real statistical freak. Such a state of fitness would be a purely temporary phenomenon because every human being faces the prospect of ageing, with its consequent decline in physical ability.

Elderly people

Myths

To be socially valued in our present society, it is necessary to be economically productive. Those who do not do paid work – housewives, the unemployed, the elderly – are consistently devalued because the protestant work ethic is alive and well in Western society. Labour is upheld for its own sake as being the factor which, above all else, gives meaning to our existence.

In terms of positive media presentation the elderly are virtually an invisible age group. The elderly who do appear in drama or comedy are rarely shown as competent characters. In print elderly women, especially, loom large as victims of mugging or other attacks, their frailty always stressed; yet in fact women over 60 are the least likely group to be victims of violent crime. The old are looked on with that blend of pity and contempt that formerly was reserved for sufferers of diseases like leprosy, setting the retired person apart from the day-to-day world, keeping him at arm's length because people do not want to be reminded of their own advancing years.

Facts

The more one looks at the subject of ageing the less it seems a matter of the passing of years than one of frame of mind. Some people never lose the spontaneity of their teenage years – others are staid, dull and boring before they are out of their twenties. Age in chronological years is simply one factor among many others, often a fairly trivial one. In the individual sense there is no such thing as old age but only individual people, each one at a point in the ageing process. Each has his own needs and wishes and has the right to decide what he wants from the remainder of his life. When one talks to elderly people it is common to learn that they feel 'exactly the same person as I was as a girl. The same thoughts and feelings, the same dreams, the same idea of myself that I've had as long as I can remember. I haven't changed.' The elderly are the same but different, they are human: they are not 'them' but 'us'.

Many people look forward to retirement not as an end but as a change of emphasis, a time when they can develop new interests and participate in community life, giving their wealth of experience and wisdom to enrich it. Others see themselves as we see them — unproductive and unimportant. They become disengaged from the affairs of the outside world because the outside world rejects them. They retreat into the narrow confines of their own unfulfilling surroundings, where they are deprived of stimulation and sense of purpose and develop a real or imagined feeling of being a burden to society. For these people, lonely and depressed, preoccupied with their own uselessness, the process of ageing tends to accelerate. They develop avoidable illness and do not seek help when necessary because they attribute their illness to ageing (Reissman, 1983).

Attitudes

Attitudes affect one's response to patients' needs and can thus influence the quality of nursing care given. Resident elderly patients often adopt whatever role is expected of them and the nurse's expectations may account for much of the eccentric, erratic and childish behaviour seen in them. For those who do not work with the elderly in areas specifically designed for their care, the impression of geriatric nursing as a clinical backwater may still persist. In England and Wales it was only in 1979 that geriatric nursing and community care became definite requirements for all basic general nursing courses. Nurses tend to express an unwillingness to work with the elderly rather than with those in other age groups (Seers, 1986). When asked if they would consider a career in geriatric nursing, Fielding (1986) found that 58 per cent of student nurses answered 'No'. There was also a feeling that time spent in geriatric nursing was time wasted in terms of one's career and in terms of energy that could be spent on those who had a chance of complete recovery. Geriatric nursing was seen as lacking in interest, variety and challenge; the speciality was described as 'depressing', 'too heavy' and 'too routine'.

Wade (1983) found in her survey of residential institutions caring for elderly people that it was not considered to be part of the duties of the staff to sit down and talk to residents, though there were exceptions. She found that the attitudes of care staff were not overly related to the particular setting. One ward sister said that 'When work permits staff could sit down and chat to patients,' but another sister said, 'From the first minute we come in we sit and chat to them'.

Visitors are another important source of communication with the elderly in care.

Some staff actively encouraged visitors by seeking to involve them in the life of the ward or home, while others were ambivalent. One matron disapproved of children coming into the home because they were noisy and 'charged about'. In contrast, another matron made great efforts to break down the barriers between staff and patients: 'All my nurses come back; they bring their children, they come home from school and wait here for mum. They go to see all the patients, sometimes bring a few flowers or sweets, sometimes patients give them sweets, the patients know all the nurses' children. But it is home, you see.' A warden of a Part III home said that young people did not come to visit the home and residents 'did not want bothering', while another described how the elderly shared their grandchildren: 'Whenever there are new babies this is one of the first places they visit' (Wade, 1983).

Epilepsy

Health care practitioners may provide excellent caring services for patients but do not care for each other. Nursing has a particularly bad record in this respect, as is seen by correspondence in the nursing press. A nurse or midwife who admits to having epilepsy will either be rejected on application or asked to leave her job, yet doctors can practise after declaring that they have an epileptic disorder.

A sister on a busy surgical ward suddenly developed epilepsy and was cruelly stigmatised by members of her own profession as well as by her medical advisers.

> Matron informed me that I was medically unfit to nurse. The doctor had interviewed my parents . . . advising my mother that I would be best living with someone who was willing to take care of me, making sure that I took the drugs at the right time and that I did not get into places which might prove dangerous should I start a fit (Campling, 1981).

Perhaps the idiocy of rejecting nurses who develop epilepsy is becoming apparent, for after a $3\frac{1}{2}$-month cessation of her employment, one nurse was offered a choice of jobs, all in nursing, through the support of her professional association (Redshaw, 1987).

French (1989) explains that 'The disabilities that people have are often used to describe them. That is, their disability is used as a noun rather than an adjective — "he's a spastic", "she's a mongol" or "he's an epileptic".' As French says: 'Language is important in the shaping of perceptions and attitudes'. By avoiding stigmatising language nurses can encourage more positive thinking about people with an epileptic disorder, be they patients or colleagues.

Pain

Nurses expect to see visible signs of pain, but in reality lack of its expression does not necessarily mean that there is none. We praise and reward the patient who tolerates pain but, in fact, this is nothing to do with bravery or cowardice, as each individual has a unique response to pain. When nurses describe a patient as having a low pain tolerance this is often accompanied by some disapproval — that the patient should be able to tolerate such an insignificant amount of pain! This value judgment interferes with a nurse's ability to provide effective intervention.

Typically, we expect that a person who complains of moderate to severe pain will exhibit the objective signs usually associated with acute pain: these include the autonomic (sympathetic) responses of elevated blood pressure, increased heart rate, rapid respiration, dilated pupils and increased perspiration. We may also expect to see the patient crying, grimacing, writhing or supporting the affected part. In the absence of these signs, the nurse may doubt that the patient's pain is moderate to severe. What she may be witnessing, however, is an adaptive response to chronic pain. The human organism is incapable of sustaining increased autonomic function indefinitely, so that although the suffering continues, the original responses may not.

A patient may complain of a level of pain higher than the nurse believes to be appropriate after a particular operation. The nurse's biases may stem from preconceived ideas of how much pain should exist with each disease entity. A patient complaining of pain may be so active and cheerful that the presence of pain is doubted by the nursing staff. Beyerman (1982) describes a woman in hospital who was visited by other patients, talked on the telephone and with her many visitors and helped to pass out water jugs, but the nurses tended to forget all about her headaches until medication time. She requested and received her medication exactly every 4 hours; she never missed a dose. It was precisely because she was so busy and involved that she was able to tolerate the pain for longer periods of time: her many activities kept her from focusing her attention on the pain − she was effectively using distraction as a method of coping with pain.

Bourbonnais (1981) has identified some areas in which nurses are not prepared to communicate with patients in their care who are in pain: personal remedies for pain are not elicited from patients, especially those with chronic pain. Some nurses give analgesics routinely with evening sedation while others wait until perhaps the patient is moaning in pain.

Sexuality

'Sexuality is a complex issue which is dependent on a number of factors such as age, culture, religion, personal experience, myths and fantasy' (Yates, 1987). The indefinable nature of human sexuality is considered by Coughlan (1987) who says that 'our sexuality encompasses many of our human qualities; it is constant and energetic and affects our physical, psychological, emotional, spiritual and social selves'. The problem of sexuality for patients has been well stated by Webb (1985): 'Communicating with [sexual] feelings verbally and non-verbally is highly problematic in hospitals and residential institutions because people are sensitive to others' reactions and afraid of embarrassment.' Coughlan (1987) explains that nurses 'may have difficulty in discussing concerns of a sexual nature because of embarrassment and inhibition'. Before the nurse can cope with the sexual needs of her patients she may need to discuss her own sexuality in supportive serious discussions with colleagues. In order to help patients Coughlan (1987) says, 'A perceptive and caring member of the health team who is constantly with the patient in whom he has confidence and trust can provide the opportunity for uninhibited discussion and reassurance about the normality of the patient's concern.' If maintaining sexuality improves the quality of life for the neurological patient, this subject can no longer remain a neglected area of patient care.

Professionalism

It may be that nurses avoid talking to patients about their fears and anxieties because they do not want to find themselves in a position where they are asked awkward questions. Sometimes, we actively discourage patients from asking questions and from seeking information. We cannot become deeply involved in the problems of our patients, yet we are not machines but human beings looking after other human beings, so that complete detachment is unacceptable. Our own experience of life and living, whether happy or sad, will, or at least should, help us to communicate more effectively with our patients. A professional attitude need not equal an unrelentingly stiff upper lip. For a few doctors the chronic patient could become the embodiment of their failure to cure, but for many nurses the chronic patient is an embodiment of their success at caring.

Chronic illness

Psychology

Every episode of physical illness has some degree of emotional significance for the patient. Not only is the individual's overall adjustment threatened but chronic illness will, at the very least, interfere with his capacity to work. This frequently results in financial difficulties and loss of self-esteem. Pain wears down the individual's defences by constantly subjecting him to unpleasant stimuli with which he is powerless to deal.

Reduced mobility results in multiple handicaps, from difficulty in performing tasks around the house to loss of employment and social contact. The effort to maintain some level of normal activity within functional limitations may be frustrating and tiring (Bury, 1982). Less obvious, but no less central to the experience of illness, are the uncertainties and worries about the prognosis of variable and fluctuating disorders such as multiple sclerosis. The fear of being different is common in those with physical abnormalities. The emotional reactions include sorrow, shame, envy, resentment, compensatory pride and sense of uniqueness and specialness, often with a sense of special power.

The personality structure of a person prior to the onset of a neurological disorder will have a profound effect on his adjustment to any physical disability. The person who feels most comfortable in a dependent relationship may find his disability a social justification for living an extremely dependent life, an answer to his psychological needs. In someone who has paranoid tendencies the disability can justify and intensify the belief that others are out to harm him. For the person who needs an isolated life-style the forced intimacy of having someone feed, bath and clothe him can be very threatening and anxiety-provoking. But the person who tends to be obsessive and compulsive may make the best adjustment because he can use these traits to cope with the tedium of self-care.

Guilt

The presence of a genetic condition in a family can lead to attitudes of crime and punishment or guilt. They may see the disease as a punishment for their sins or even for sins committed in the distant past by their ancestors. People who have seen a parent deteriorate with Huntington's chorea may feel guilty about the anger they feel toward him or worry that they have neglected him. Childless women are faced with the choice of guilt or self-deprivation. The traditionally negative associations around the epilepsies causes guilt in parents who worry about what they may have wrongly done that has caused the disorder. The term 'stroke' derives from the ancient belief that it occurred as a stroke 'from above', a punishment for some misdeed, and the passive response of patients and their relatives who wait and see what happens in the following few days may be related to this.

Caring produces guilty feelings about not doing the job to perfection. The carer may at times wish that she might die so she would not have to cope any longer and later experience awful guilt at the thought. Family members report feelings of frustration and guilt concerning an angry thought or response to the irritating behaviour of a demented spouse or parent. The carer's guilt is compounded by the patient's own guilt at being a 'burden' on his family and from the effect of his suffering on people close to him. Guilt is not inevitable: it can be avoided by striking a realistic balance between the needs of the carer and those of the dependant. The balance will bring a rewarding and happy relationship.

An unfortunate consequence of public education campaigns about acquired immune deficiency (AIDS) is the implication that if people get AIDS in the future, it will be their own fault. Knowledge about lengthy incubation periods can be conveniently ignored when people wish to attribute blame to those whose life-style is considered to be the greatest risk factor in their acquiring the disease.

The family

A family consists of individuals who interact but can be recognised as an entity: the whole is greater than the parts. If one member changes, some compensatory change must occur in the rest of the family, and if the role of that individual is seriously altered, this may require a complete reorganisation of family life. Incapacity of the breadwinner, in particular, may lead to a reduction of the family's standard of living. All the family will have to cope with anxiety, anger, guilt and sadness.

Marriage

A neurological disorder can cause considerable unhappiness within the family, especially between marriage partners. If the basic relationship is poor the neurological disorder may be made the scapegoat for all marital or sexual problems and may lead to separation or divorce. Some sufferers fall readily into the sick role, which they use to manipulate their partners or other relatives by inducing guilty feelings, while others deny the disease so much that they refuse to acknowledge any limitations. Life then becomes difficult for all members of the family in different ways. Marriage partners may find it difficult to express feelings of anger, which can lead to lack of communication and misunderstanding. If the bond between two people is sufficiently strong and based upon values and interests that are not just transitory, marriage to someone who has a neurological disorder can be a great success despite the difficulties.

A further complication of family relationships may be the process of regression that many disabled people undergo. The need for love and comfort from the soothing touch of a loved one is often difficult to request or is withheld for fear that the injured person will feel babied. Part of the resistance to requesting physical comforting is the fear of revulsion that the disabled person feels toward his own body and which he may expect others also to feel. If the sense of revulsion is severely felt, the person also begins to fear abandonment, projecting the sense of a lack of ability to deal with his changed body onto family members or a sexual partner.

Dependence

Mature dependence is a relationship involving evenly matched giving and taking between two individuals who are mutually dependent. Even if a disabled person is physically dependent, his emotional strengths may lead others to depend on him. Nurses may find this when working in a residential community where residents and staff consult the most physically disabled person for advice and encouragement. Such mutual interdependence should be acknowledged, whether it occurs in hospital or in the family situation.

People react differently to the problem of physical dependence. Nevertheless, one reason why some, perhaps the majority, resent it is the feeling of obligation and of a difference in status that arises from being always on the receiving end. To call attention to themselves, to stand out in the crowd by having to ask for help, is a fear that many disabled people discuss with nurses. It tends to make them feel that they belong to a minority group and, even more, to a socially inferior minority group, so that help is frequently rejected for this reason. The disabled person has to resolve the conflict between two antagonistic situations: the desire to achieve maximum independence and to be treated as anyone else, but requiring help that others do not need.

If a family incorrectly perceives that illness causes a member to be different rather than just to act differently on occasion, they may believe him to be more dependent than he is. The overprotective parents who live in dread of their child dying or being injured during a fit may raise an angry, resentful young adult who has to make a supreme effort to find his own identity.

Disabled people may be physically dependent on others in ways that range from minimal assistance to total care. Those people who need help with toilet and menstrual care, or with feeding, usually find the necessity for such intimate care very difficult to accept because of its association with babyhood, while the help that some disabled people require in meeting their sexual needs may diminish their feelings of masculinity or femininity. When a disabled person is always dependent on others, whether this dependence is physical, financial or emotional, he experiences feelings of obligation and stigma – feelings of being in the power of another, of being dominated. Dysphasia puts a great strain on marital relationships.

Leisure

It does not take much imagination to understand how social relationships are disrupted, or falter and disintegrate under the stress of a neurological disorder. The state of chronic dependency leads to feelings of frustration, of unworthiness or alienation and low self-esteem, and the patient may cultivate a studiously ignorant and deferential helplessness.

Reduced mobility, difficulty in communicating and problems with hearing or vision all tend to place restrictions on an individual's ability to retain old friendships as well as establish new ones. Maintaining normal activities, for example being able to sit in one position for a long period of time at a cinema, or maintaining normal appearances in a social gathering at a club or pub, have to become deliberately conscious activities and thus frustrating and tiring. In the end the effort simply does not seem worth it: the simplest outing becomes a major occasion of planning and expedition. The individual begins to restrict his terrain to local and familial territory where he is least likely to be exposed to the gaze and questions of acquaintances and strangers.

Brain damage

When a person has sustained brain damage he becomes dependent on his family for self-care and the daily activities of cooking and housekeeping. People who have had a stroke (CVA) will reduce their social contacts and leisure activities even when there has only been minimal disability; this also happens in the younger person who has had a head injury. Possible reasons for this altered social life are personality and cognitive changes, in particular memory changes.

One study compared the social effect upon their wives of soldiers who suffered either a penetrating brain injury or paraplegia. The wives of the brain-injured soldiers suffered a greater reduction in social activities than the wives of paraplegics. These wives felt that their husbands' condition was a social handicap and also considered that their friends were deserting them (Rosenbaum and Najenson, 1976). The spouses of patients who have had a stroke appear to have similar experiences to wives of men with a head injury. The reduction in leisure activities, contacts with friends and other social contacts is experienced most acutely by those whose spouse is dysphasic (Kinsella and Duffy, 1979).

Parkinson's disease

Problems with daily activities were reported by people who answered a questionnaire sent to members of the Parkinson's Disease Society: 83 per cent (216) had difficulty with writing, 67 per cent (174) with managing buttons and zips in dressing and 63 per cent (164) with turning over in bed. Bathing, getting into and out of bed or a chair were difficult tasks for more than half of the respondents. Constipation was by far the most common complaint, dry mouth the second most common, and involuntary movements associated with dopaminergic drugs the third. It was in the younger age group where the sufferer had to give up work that families most frequently perceived themselves as suffering economic hardship, because of the disparity between expected and actual income (Gibberd, 1985; Nanton, 1985; Singer, 1973).

Multiple sclerosis

In an attempt to evaluate the consequences of a disabling illness, people with multiple sclerosis were asked to keep a diary. In contrast to the general population, the multiple sclerosis group took rests during the day, at 7.30 a.m. just before getting up, at 2.30 p.m. and at 10 p.m. when they were awake but in bed before falling asleep. Time spent 'sitting' is also much higher with multiple sclerosis than in the general population. Women with multiple sclerosis who spent more time caring for children than did others described this activity as the compensation they felt for their perceived inadequacies as mothers in other respects. They also concentrated more on one activity at a time than did other women (Lawson et al, 1985).

Gilles de la Tourette syndrome

The Gilles de la Tourette syndrome inflicts great damage on sufferers, who experience feelings of isolation and loneliness. Trying to maintain control over the symptoms can be exhausting and destructive to interpersonal relationships. Involuntary movements have to be altered to look purposeful, so what started as involuntary is developed into a gesture of fanning oneself, coughing or stretching. The fear of being isolated and alone can be very disturbing. One young man said he had abandoned the possibility of a mutually satisfying relationship as he felt that no-one would be able to tolerate his movements.

The carers

When a person experiences a neurological disorder that involves both physical and mental changes, this requires a big adjustment by the closest relatives and friends: thus, not only is the pattern of the relationship altered but its very quality may be changed. There may be a deterioration in parent–child relationships following a stroke (CVA) in a parent. A man who has always led an independent life may find it difficult to accept a dependent role, as indeed may his partner.

Women seem more likely to take on the entire responsibility of care-giving and are more reluctant to ask for help. Tyler (1987) endorsed earlier findings that the majority (60 per cent) of carers are women, although the number of men caring for elderly spouses was shown to be 38 per cent, with a further 2 per cent caring for other relatives.

Many people who have had a stroke and are left disabled for months or years are cared for by their family, at great cost: half suffer financial stress; three-quarters have a loss of social life; 60 per cent have disrupted sleep. Caring for a stroke survivor increases the carer's risk of anxiety for 6 months and depression for 1 year after the event. By 2 years, depression in the carers was not related to their worries about the condition of the stroke victim (Wade et al, 1986).

Sharing caring

A single carer should not try to carry the whole load of the illness on his or her shoulders. The Alzheimer's Disease Society offers sound advice to carers: 'Looking after yourself involves sharing the care of the patient, so that you have time to maintain interests' (ADS, 1984). They suggest that a family meeting should be arranged in order to allocate clear responsibilities, preferably with help from a counsellor. Some family members may simply not realise what the carer is experiencing or may not be aware of fairly easy ways in which they could help. Relatives may keep away because of their own feelings of sadness at the deterioration of the patient. Small children frequently relate very well to dementing older people and are able to establish special and loving relationships with them – they can be encouraged to visit and play with the patient.

Different family members and, when possible, friends outside the immediate household should take turns to spend time with the dysphasic patient. In this way no individual member of the family will be overburdened and the patient will be given adequate opportunity to relearn how to communicate with a variety of companions. Even if the patient finds communicating difficult, he should remain within the family group and be allowed to be present when friends visit. If he is deprived of these social contacts, his ultimate ability to recover understanding and to communicate properly will be delayed or rendered impossible (Cooper, 1976).

There is a tendency for care-givers to become quite isolated, receiving fewer and fewer visits from friends and going out less frequently. The timely use of home helps and day centres can considerably reduce the stress for the care-giver and delay premature institutionalisation of the affected person. In some situations, the care-giver will be fortunate enough to have someone to talk to when upset or troubled. A family member will sometimes undertake this role, but as many families have no history of confiding in one another a counsellor or support group might satisfy this need.

In a study of alternative provision of care for elderly people, which gave the regular carer(s) temporary relief from the sole responsibility of caring, Tyler (1987) found that the satisfaction with individual types of respite care provision varied immensely: 74.4 per cent found it very effective in reducing stress for them; 15.3 per cent found that it helped a little. Many carers made urgent and poignant pleas for more respite care in the elderly person's usual home, suggesting an extension of existing sitting and home help/domiciliary care assistant schemes. The need for relief care at night was emphasised by carers, some suggesting the extended use of existing day care provision, many feeling that the current provision of night sitters was a most successful way of providing this type of respite care but wishing it could be extended to cover more nights.

Relatives' questions

When relatives of a dementing patient ask whether or not his condition will worsen, they are raising one of the most disturbing issues that must be faced. They do not know for how long the problem will go on, or what to expect next. Carers have to look honestly and realistically at what the future holds for them and the patient. Nobody wants to think about a sad future and not looking too far ahead is often a natural way of getting on with life. However, ignoring things that must be faced and coped with in these circumstances is costly in the end. The dementing patient will be able to do fewer and fewer things and become less and less able to communicate verbally. Eventually there may be deep confusion, incontinence and immobility. At the same time, the patient will become more and more vulnerable to illnesses such as pneumonia and other infections (ADS, 1984).

It has been suggested by Stevens (1982) that families should be warned that the patient with Huntington's chorea might have psychiatric symptoms, which could lead to difficulties later on, so the problems can be anticipated and the distress averted. The patient's friends and workmates may have to be told that he is ill to prevent these people from concluding that the choreic is constantly drunk: this common misinterpretation of the symptoms can cause much distress.

In discussing 'the forgotten sufferers' the Alzheimer's Disease Society (ADS, 1984) asks:

> How long can the family accept the responsibility of care? With advancing disease, there may come a time when people are less important to the patient than the service they give. It may no longer matter who gives the service as long as it is done; there may be no longer true recognition or special reaction to a loved one. Physical needs and their satisfaction are the only things that matter. At this point one must ask the question, 'Is this situation manageable?'

Many questions put to the nurse by relatives will be direct requests for support and encouragement: skill in responding to questions may depend more on the attitudes and values of people with whom she works than on special courses that she may have attended.

The professionals

The first error is to decide that, as nurses, we know what would be best for the family, and to tell them what to do, without considering their needs or wishes. Behaviour varies to too great an extent, as do the values and resources of families, to apply one approach as the 'right' one. The second error is to assume that when they seek help families have enough information on which to decide what they want.

The most important consideration in relating to dementing patients is to treat them with dignity. Even when they do not understand or respond, it is better to assume that they understand at least something about the situation: they may respond to the emotional connotations of a situation, rather than the overt, but in this way they do maintain some relationship with their family. Patients often appear to know the attitudes of people who interact with them, whether those people are friendly or hostile, sympathetic or angry (Zarit, 1985).

Stigma

Culture

The dominant view of disability is one of personal tragedy or disaster but this varies in different societies. Variations in the cultural view of disability are not just a random matter but may occur as a result of a number of factors such as the type of economy and the social structure and values of a society. A hierarchical structure like that in Britain, which is based upon values of individual success through personal achievement, inevitably means that most disabled people are well down in the hierarchy on the basis of their reduced ability to compete on equal terms with everyone else. Societies whose central values are religious may well interpret disability as punishment for sin or possession by the devil, or as a sign of being chosen by God. In short, 'disability' does not have a similar meaning in all cultures nor, indeed, within the same culture is there always agreement about what disability actually is. Heroic figures in classical children's literature are usually described in terms of physical perfection. Bad people have peg-legs, facial disfigurement or an eyepatch, whereas virtue is rewarded with physical grace. The ugly duckling turns into a swan, the frog becomes a king and the beast changes into a prince. This trend is also found in adult literature, although in more subtle forms. From the Bible through Sophocles, Chaucer, Shakespeare, Dostoevsky and Dickens, characters who are disabled and good are difficult to find. When a disabled person is good he is portrayed in the arts as supergood, superstrong and supercourageous.

Stigma

The word *stigma* refers to the disgrace associated with certain conditions, attributes, traits, or forms of behaviour. In the case of the chronically ill this marking may be an obvious deformity, ungainly or uncoordinated movements, or the necessity to use the paraphernalia of disability such as sticks, crutches or wheelchairs.

Labels

There are many words or labels within the English language that evoke immediate mental stereotypes and assumptions about the person to whom the label is attached: for example, Irish, woman, elderly, mental, subnormal, retarded, teenager, unemployed. It is commonly accepted that to be elderly means to be unintelligent, unemployable, probably mentally disturbed, incontinent, feeble and asexual. Sutherland (1981) explains how the term 'the disabled' depersonalises and writes off people with disabilities as individuals by implying that their disabilities are their identity. He says, 'The disabled are generally understood to be a small, clearly defined section of society, quite distinct from the public at large – poor dependent creatures, immediately recognisable as physically different from normal people.' The change from the 'disabled' to 'people with disabilities' was not a plea against the disability but against depersonalisation and the right to make 'person' the core of the phrase. The nurse who refers to a patient as epileptic is taking one feature of the patient to characterise him as a whole. Consequently, the individual stops being a person or someone who may need special consideration some of the time and becomes a disabled person, identified solely by his medical problem and the limitations it imposes.

Another way in which disabled patients are stigmatised is when any difficulty they may have with some of the activities of everyday living is generalised by the non-disabled to *all* activities, whether physical or cognitive. Locker (1983) provides some crude examples of such stigma:

> There were a group of us, some had MS and some had other things and we were sitting next to these people and they said 'Excuse me asking but which home are you from?' I said 'My own.' She gives me a look and I say 'And so are they.' And as I turned away I heard her say 'I thought they were all from some mental institution.' But I didn't enlighten her, I just said 'my own home' and left it at that.

A more subtle form of this assumption of incompetence is the 'Does he take sugar?' syndrome in which it is assumed that disabled people are incapable of responding to questions about their capacities and needs. 'I had to go round to the solicitor to have an affidavit sworn and he came out to the car and said "Can you write?"'

Visibility

Whether or not a disabled person will be helped and accepted or confined and isolated depends on the severity of the disability, the degree to which its course can be predicted and controlled, the visibility of the handicap and the fear it produces in the onlooker. Locker (1983) found that people with rheumatoid arthritis were able to conceal their condition most of the time. Those who presented accounts of stigmatising encounters tended to be those who used wheelchairs or had a visible physical deformity. For them, their impairment and disability often became the central focus of interaction with the non-disabled. Some people may be stigmatised more by the consequences of a disorder, for example, unemployment and poverty, than by the disorder itself.

Communication

Healthy people tend to stand further away from disabled people during interaction, to end conversations with them sooner than they do with other normal healthy people and to feel less comfortable emotionally in interaction with the physically disabled. It is as though a deformed and paralysed body attacks everyone's sense of well-being and invincibility. Most people prefer to avoid those who are sick or old as they are disturbing reminders of unwelcome reality.

Relatives of disabled people may find it difficult to express or even feel anger towards the person who has the disability, regardless of how irritating such a person's personality can be or how offensive his behaviour. As the non-disabled tend to feel it necessary to watch their every gesture and word closely in order not to make a negative slip or show their aversion, and because norms regulating disabled and non-disabled interaction are quite ambiguous for both parties, such interactions are reported as uncomfortable, rigid and strained.

When the health condition is in doubt greater problems in interpersonal relationships seem to arise. Relatives wonder if the patient is malingering in order to get attention, which can cause strained relations. For an individual with an invisible stigma information management is a matter of concern – how much should he reveal about himself and to whom? Some physically disabled people may almost be ostracised, for which there are two main reasons: one is that disability may make them embarrassed or uncertain how to behave, so they tend to avoid a situation which makes them feel uncomfortable; a second reason is fear, the fear that able-bodied relatives or friends may have of becoming involved, practically and emotionally, in a situation where there is no clear ending to the commitment. Also, the sight of the physical limitations of a disabled person may arouse the conscious fear in able-bodied people that they themselves may at some time become equally disabled.

Motivation, physical incapacity and impairment make a difference in human interaction. An individual with a visible stigma may be handicapped by uncertainty when engaging in social contacts with unstigmatised individuals: wondering what the other is thinking of him; feeling self-conscious about the impression he is making; guarding against exaggerated perceptions of his accomplishments, as well as his weaknesses, are among his key activities.

A chronically ill person usually presents different techniques of adapting to his situation, depending on the relationships involved. Someone with no striking evidence of multiple sclerosis may pass as well to strangers. However, to family members that person may be viewed as sick and may be allowed certain privileges, such as exemption from household chores. Friends may see him as being well but feigning sickness in order to get attention.

The physically disabled person may feel shame as he tries to manage his spoiled identity; the physically normal person also feels discomfort and may then reject and withdraw from encounters with the physically deviant (Goffman, 1968). When a person is attempting to pass as normal, the emphasis is on concealing some aspect of his identity from other people in order to avoid the negative, condescending and deprecating attitudes of others. The psychological costs of using this strategy are high: if the concealment is discovered, the person may be embarrassed or humiliated, friendships may be destroyed, or a job lost (e.g. in epilepsy).

Self-esteem

Self-acceptance involves the ability to view oneself honestly and acknowledge one's many shortcomings, and yet to live happily and creatively with this awareness free of undue anxiety, self-criticism or defensive compensations. Much of what a person chooses to do and the manner in which he does it is presumed to be dependent upon his self-esteem. A person's evaluation or esteem of himself plays a key role in determining his behaviour.

In general, high self-esteem is associated with good adjustment and little anxiety, insecurity or defensiveness. In contrast to this, people with low self-esteem are more likely to exhibit anxiety and neurotic behaviour, to perform less effectively under stress and to be socially ineffective overall. People who usually display extremes of behaviour are seldom well-adjusted, and a moderate self-esteem level represents a balance between self-criticism and self-enhancement.

Wexler (1979) reported that no matter how mature and well-adjusted men and women 'at risk' were to the presence of Huntington's chorea in the family, the nature of the symptoms seemed to strike at the core of their physical and psychological self-esteem. Subjects spoke repeatedly of how 'disgusting', 'repulsive', 'grotesque', 'ugly and horrible' the Huntington's patient becomes. There was a particular dread of losing bladder and bowel control. Some reported feeling nauseated at the sight of their ill parents.

Epilepsy

Many people with epilepsy are resentful or embarrassed about their seizure disorder and find themselves ill at ease at the possibility of seizures. They feel that they are less worthwhile and less accepted by others because of the seizures. The person with repeated seizures may begin to lose his self-esteem if others continue to reject him (Ozuna, 1979). As the patient sees it, the consequences of having epilepsy are distorted by misconception, ignorance or mood disorder, or through misunderstanding by others. Many patients carry erroneous beliefs about epilepsy and suffer from some of the kinds of misinformation and prejudice seen in the general population. The primary factor influencing the patient's social and psychological status is his own, along with his relatives', perception of the epilepsy: people with epilepsy tend to regard themselves as less well endowed.

One study found that people with epilepsy evaluated themselves frequently as depressed and fearful and that they tended to hide their anger. Of the 60 people interviewed, 30 per cent felt themselves to be rejected and only 25 per cent believed that they were totally accepted by others. People whose epilepsy was identified in early childhood had a low self-esteem, in contrast to people whose epileptic disorder started later in life. The people who had lived with an epileptic disorder all their lives tended to be resigned to it and accepted it in a fatalistic way (Janzik et al, 1978).

The patient may be prevented from developing individuality and self-esteem by an overprotective family. A family's 'felt' stigma can lead to eroded self-image. Patients may have their morale and self-esteem destroyed by their family's attitude of unacceptability, disapproval and rejection. Someone with repeated seizures who begins to lose self-esteem if others continue to reject him may become withdrawn from society in order to avoid the unpleasant reactions of others.

Employment

It is of fundamental importance to pay attention to the patient's own motivation and his opinion of his own capabilities. A person's observations of how others react to him modifies all his internal psychological processes: the sense of self. To succeed in employment, people need to be highly motivated and have self-confidence, a good verbal IQ and the ability to socialise. It is common for patients who have failed to establish themselves socially or at work to attribute their failure to other people's prejudice. Too often problems of those with epilepsy are presented as factors over which they have no control, and they are presented as the passive recipients of many injustices. The world must change in order to make those with epilepsy more comfortable (McGuckin, 1980).

The situation of people with epilepsy is characterised less by the experience of actual stigmatisation than by a largely false belief that others hold negative attitudes and are ever ready to discriminate. Scambler and Hopkins (1986) investigated the impact of epilepsy on 94 people on the lists of 17 GPs in and around London. They found that although almost all those with epilepsy who had worked full-time believed epilepsy to be stigmatising, only 23 per cent could recall a single occasion when they suspected they had been victims of actual stigma at work, even of casual ridicule. Fourteen per cent reported episodes that, in their judgment, had inhibited their careers in some way.

This study showed that more unhappiness, anxiety and self-doubt was caused by the fear of stigma than either directly or indirectly through actual stigma. Most full-time workers were found to be on guard against being identified as having epilepsy and some had also denied themselves opportunities of career advancement. Worries about stigma led married women with husbands in secure employment to abandon plans for making their own careers. The authors concluded that the fear of stigma and shame associated with being epileptic 'is more disruptive of the lives of people with epilepsy than enacted stigma'. If the public has become better informed and less intolerant about epilepsy than formerly, nurses should be more optimistic and help patients to aim for a full, satisfying life-style.

Immobility

Besides problems of attitude, the relative social isolation of disabled people is partly due to problems of mobility, which affect access and the use of public transport. The ways in which the health and welfare services are organised tend to segregate disabled people and to separate them further from social contacts with able-bodied people in the community.

Various body parts that are affected by a disabling condition can have specific psychological significance for the individual. Paralysis of the lower limbs can revive earlier feelings about separation and independence experienced by the child learning to walk. The wheelchair-bound person who must always look up at people can be affected by the question of mastery and size. Paralysis of the upper limbs can plunge the person into the total dependency of the new-born, where he needs someone to feed, clothe and bathe him. These body changes necessitate changes in the person's self-image and this may be compounded by the need also to assimilate foreign objects, such as aids to mobility, into the sense of self.

Involuntary movements

Many patients firmly date the onset of tremor to a particularly distressing personal event such as bereavement, a business setback or an accident. The importance of emotional factors in enhancing latent tremor cannot be denied but this does not mean that they cause the symptom. Because it attracts attention and is difficult to conceal, a tremor can be troublesome. The more a person tries to prevent people noticing it, the more nervous and tense he becomes and embarrassment makes the tremor difficult to control. Patients have to learn to live with a tremor because medical treatment will not suppress it completely.

The most difficult aspect of suffering from an involuntary movement is that people will stare and ridicule the possessor of an attribute that deviates from normal behaviour and is therefore seen to be unnatural and deeply discrediting. People with dyskinesia are convinced that others will interpret their movements as a sign of mental illness: it is the visibility of the symptoms that makes them distressing. Patients who have had Gilles de la Tourette syndrome since childhood feel frustrated in trying to overcome the social restrictions they have felt as a result of the reaction of people to the disorder.

Facial disfigurement

The face is the source of vocal communication, the expressor of emotions and the revealer of personality traits. The face is the person himself. A facial disfigurement is more of a social handicap than a physical one. This is because suffering results from the visibility of the defect and the person is handicapped because of his appearance. Reactions to facially deformed people may include staring, remarks, curiosity, questioning, pity, rejection, ridicule, whispering, nicknames and discrimination. The twisted mouth, inappropriate grimaces and movements of the head may well be a barrier to the privileges and opportunities available to people without such visible disabilities.

Patients' experiences

Mary, who suffered from tardive dyskinesia, was convinced that they were staring at her. Her hands were so shaky that with each sip the coffee spilled on her hands and clothes. She peered around the coffee shop. Yes, they were watching every move she made. Suddenly her jaw began to jerk from side to side and she bit her tongue. Her neck began to extend backwards and the muscles of her face started to twitch. She quickly left the shop and ran back to the privacy of her room at home.

Another example of an embarrassing movement disorder is in the victim of Huntington's chorea whose facial muscles

—twitched and contorted, giving him a strange, grotesque grimace. He had difficulty eating without spilling his food. Worst of all, he realised that his appearance was abhorrent to other people. When they recoiled in his presence, he tried to hide it. He wanted to stay away from other people as much as he could (Phillips, 1982).

Using a wheelchair can stir up primitive fears in onlookers.

She was pushing him in his wheelchair through the narrow streets of a small market town when they met an old woman draped in a long black shawl. The woman was dismayed by what she saw, for she seemed to look anxiously about her as if hunting for an escape route. Not finding one she had to pass close to the fearful object in her path. She made a religious sign as if to protect herself from the evil eye and then as she went by, she slipped him a few coins before hurrying away! (Burnfield, 1985).

References

ADS (1984) *Caring For The Person with Dementia*. London: Alzheimer's Disease Society.

Beyerman K (1982) Flawed perceptions about pain. *American Journal of Nursing*, **82**(2): 302–304.

Bourbonnais F (1981) Pain assessment: development of a tool for the nurse and the patient. *Journal of Advanced Nursing*, **6**(4): 277–282.

Burnfield A (1985) *Multiple Sclerosis: A Personal Exploration*. London: Souvenir Press.

Bury M (1982) Chronic illness as biographical disruption. *Sociology of Health and Illness*, **4**(2): 167–182.

Campbell-Hayes C (1988) Presidential address. *Assistant Librarian*, **81**(7): 105–109.

Campling J (ed.) (1981) *Images of Ourselves*. London: Routledge and Kegan Paul.

Cooper I S (1976) *Living with Neurological Disease: A Handbook For The Patient and The Family*. New York: Norton and Co.

Coughlan (1987) Dear nurse. *Nursing Times*, **85**(42): 32–34.

Coughlan A and Humphrey M (1982) Presenile stroke: long term outcome for patients and their families. *Rheumatology and Rehabilitation*, **21**: 115–122.

Downie P A (ed.) (1986) *Cash's Textbook on Neurology for Physiotherapists*, 4th edn. London: Faber and Faber.

Fielding P (1986) *Attitudes Revisited: An Examination of Student Nurses' Attitudes Towards Old People in Hospital*. London: Royal College of Nursing.

Frankel M, Cummings J L, Robertson M M, Trimble M R, Hill M A and Benson D F (1986) Obsessions and compulsions in Gilles de la Tourette's syndrome. *Neurology*, **36**(3): 378–382.

French S (1989) Mind yur language. *Nursing Times*, **85**(2): 29–31.

Gibberd F B, Oxtoby M and Jewell P F (1985) The treatment of Parkinson's disease – a consumer view. *Health Trends*, **17**(1): 19–21.

Goffman E (1968) *Stigma: Notes on the Management of Spoiled Identity*. Harmondsworth: Penguin.

Janzik H H, Schmitz I, Geiger G and Mayer K (1978) Correlation between epilepsy, self-esteem and social and professional factors. In: *Advances in Epileptology*, Meinardi H and Rowan A J (eds.), pp. 72–76. Amsterdam: Zwets and Zeitlinger.

Kinsella G J and Duffy F D (1979) Psychosocial readjustment in the spouses of aphasic patients. *Scandinavian Journal of Rehabilitation Medicine*, **11**: 129–132.

Lawson A, Robinson L and Bakes C (1985) Problems in evaluating the consequences of disabling illness: the case of multiple sclerosis. *Psychological Medicine*, **15**(3): 555–579.

Lishman W A (1987) *Organic Psychiatry: the Psychological Consequences of Cerebral Disorder*, 2nd edn. Oxford: Blackwell Scientific.

Locker D (1983) *Disability and Disadvantage: the Consequences of Chronic Illness*. London: Tavistock.

McGuckin H M (1980) Changing the world view of those with epilepsy. In: *Advances in Epileptology: XIth Epilepsy International Symposium*, pp. 205–208. New York: Raven Press.

Nanton V (1985) The consequences of Parkinson's disease – needs, provisions and initiatives. *Journal of Royal Society of Health*, **105**(2): 52–54.

Newman S (1984) The social and emotional consequences of head injury and stroke. *International Review of Applied Psychology*, **33**: 427–455.

Ozuna J (1979) Psychosocial aspects of epilepsy. *Journal of Neurosurgical Nursing*, **11**(4): 242–246.

Payne T (1976) Sexuality of nurses: correlations of knowledge, attitudes and behaviour. *Nursing Research*, **25**(4): 286–292.

Phillips D H (1982) *Living with Huntington's Disease: A Book for Patients and Families*. London: Junction Books.

Redshaw A (1987) Safe to nurse. *Lampada*, **10**: 20–21.

Reissman H (1983) Make a conscious effort. *Nursing Mirror*, **157**(24): 36–37.

Robinson R and Price T (1982) Post stroke depressive disorders: a follow-up of 103 patients. *Stroke*, **13**(5): 635–641.

Rosenbaum M and Najenson T (1976) Changes in life patterns and symptoms of low mood as reported by wives of severely brain-injured soldiers. *Journal of Consulting and Clinical Psychology*, **44**: 881–888.

Sacks O (1987) *A Leg To Stand On*. New York: Harper and Row.

Salter M (ed.) (1988) *Altered Body Image – The Nurse's Role*. Chichester: John Wiley and Sons.

Scambler G and Hopkins A (1986) Being epileptic: coming to terms with stigma. *Sociology of Health and Illness*, **8**(1): 26–43.

Scheinberg I and Sternlieb I (1984) *Wilson's Disease*. Philadelphia: W B Saunders.

Seers C (1986) Talking to the elderly and its relevance to care. *Nursing Times* Occasional Paper, **82**(1): 51–54.

Singer E (1973) Social costs of Parkinson's disease. *Journal of Chronic Diseases*, **26**: 243–244.

Stevens D L (1982) *Huntington's Chorea*. Leicestershire: Association to Combat Huntington's Chorea.

Sutherland A T (1981) *Disabled We Stand*, p. 13. London: Souvenir Press.

Tyler J (1987) Give us a break. *Nursing Times*, **83**(50): 32–35.

Wade B (1983) Different models of care for the elderly. *Nursing Times* Occasional Paper, **79**(12): 33–36.

Wade D T, Leigh-Smith J and Langton-Hewer R (1986) Effects of living and looking after survivors of a stroke. *British Medical Journal*, **293**(2): 418–420.

Webb C (1985) *Sexuality, Nursing and Health*, pp. 70–71. Chichester: John Wiley and Sons.

Wexler N S (1979) Genetic 'Russian roulette'. The experience of being 'at risk' for Huntington's disease. In: *Genetic Counselling Psychological Dimensions*, Kessler S (ed.) pp. 201–202. Academic Press.

Yates A (1987) And baby makes three . . . . *Nursing Times*, **12**(83): 31–34.

Zarit S H, Orr N K and Zarit J M (1985) *The Hidden Victims of Alzheimer's Disease: Families under Stress*. New York: New York University Press.

Further reading

Feelings of patients and relatives

Beckenham M (1986) Patients' points of view. *Senior Nurse*, **4**(3): 26–27.

Bridges K W and Goldberg D P (1984) Psychiatric illness in patients with neurological disorders: patients' views on discussion of emotional problems with neurologists. *British Medical Journal*, **289**(2): 656–658.

Briggs A and Oliver J (eds.) (1985) *Caring; Experiences of Looking after Disabled Relatives*. London: Routledge and Kegan Paul.

Brunning B and Huffington C (1985) Altered images. *Nursing Times*, **81**(31): 24–27.

Equal Opportunities Commission (1980) *The Experience of Caring for Elderly and Handicapped Dependants: Survey Report*. Manchester: Equal Opportunities Commission.

Gloag D (1985) Epilepsy and employment. *British Medical Journal*, **192**(1): 2–3.

Goodman C (1986) Research on the informal carer: a selected literature review. *Journal of Advanced Nursing*, **11**(6): 705–712.

Jones D A, Victor C A and Vetter N J (1984) Hearing difficulty and its psychological implications for the elderly. *Journal of Epidemiology and Community Health*, **38**(1): 75–78.

Robinson W (1985) Foundation for living. *Senior Nurse*, **3**(2): 35–38.

Young M (1984) The expectations of patients. *Self Health*, **5**: 13–15.

Oliver J (1985) Who cares for the carers? *Self Health*, **8**: 16.

Nurses' attitudes

Alderman C (1985) Ministering angels. *Nursing Times*, **81**(21): 26–27.

Astrom S (1986) Health care students' attitudes towards, and intention to work with, patients suffering from senile dementia. *Journal of Advanced Nursing*, **11**(6): 651–659.

Benson E R (1982) Attitudes toward the elderly: a survey of recent nursing literature. *Journal of Gerontological Nursing*, **8**(2): 279–281.

Downie-Wamboldt B L and Melanson P M (1985) A descriptive study of the attitudes of baccalaureate student nurses toward the elderly. *Journal of Advanced Nursing*, **10**(4): 369–374.

Fox C (1986) Judge not . . . . *Journal of District Nursing*, **5**(4): 12, 15.

Marshall P D (1985) Nursing patients – an enjoyable task? *Journal of Advanced Nursing*, **10**(6): 429–434.

Sanderson E (1985) Nursing patience. *Lampada*, **4**: 36–37.

Snape J (1986) Nurses' attitudes to care of the elderly. *Journal of Advanced Nursing*, **11**(5): 569–572.

Wright E S (1986) Appraisal methods: how do you rate yourself? *Professional Nurse*, **1**(4): 102–104.

Chronic illness

Charmaz K (1983) Loss of self: a fundamental form of suffering in the chronically ill. *Sociology of Health and Illness*, **5**(2): 168–193.

Clough N (1984) A short answer to long-term care. *Nursing Times*, **80**(49): 40–42.

Coe R (1983) Put yourself in my place. *Nursing Mirror*, **157**(4): 48–49.

Craig H M and Edwards J E (1983) Adaptation in chronic illness; an eclectic model for nurses. *Journal of Advanced Nursing*, **8**(5): 397–404.

Dell E M (1981) *What of My Future? Re-employment of Disabled Professional People*. London: Disabled Living Foundation.

Evans R L, Becker V and Stone B W (1982) Identifying social needs of patients with neuromuscular disorders. *Rehabilitation Nursing*, Sept–Oct: 21–23, 45.

Felton B J, Revenson T A and Hinrichsen G A (1984) Stress and coping in the explanation of psychological adjustment among chronically ill adults. *Social Science and Medicine*, **18**(10): 889–898.

Hardiker P and Tod V (1982) Social work and chronic illness. *British Journal of Social Work*, **12**: 639–667.

Manpower Services Commission (1984) *Code of Good Practice on the Employment of Disabled People.* Sheffield: Manpower Services Commission.

Miller J F (ed.) (1983) *Coping With Chronic Illness.* Philadelphia: F A Davis.

Peroni F (1981) The status of chronic illness. *Social Policy and Administration,* **15**(1): 43–53.

Salter B, Battle S and Moran-Ellis J (1986) Where the buck stops. *Nursing Times,* **82**(1) *Community Outlook,* January: 19–20.

Thomas G B (1986) An unwelcome companion. *Nursing Times,* **82**(48): 36–37.

Viney L L and Westbrook M T (1984) Coping with chronic illness: strategy preferences, changes in preferences and associated emotional reactions. *Journal of Chronic Diseases,* **37**(6): 489–502.

Stigma of disability

Albrecht G, Walker V and Levy J (1982) Social distance from the stigmatized: a test of two theories. *Social Science & Medicine,* **16**: 1319–1327.

Blaxter M (1976) *The Meaning of Disability.* London: Heinemann.

Britten N, Wadsworth M E J and Fenwick P B C (1984) Stigma in patients with early epilepsy: a national longitudinal study. *Journal of Epidemiology and Community Health,* **38**(4): 291–295.

Caveness W F, Merritt H H and Galup G H (1974) A survey of public attitudes toward epilepsy in 1974 with an indication of trends over the past twenty-five years. *Epilepsia,* **15**: 523–526.

Craig A G (1980) Wasted skills and epilepsy: intervention for prevention. *Royal Society of Health Journal,* **6**: 224–226.

Dartington T, Miller E and Gwynne G (1981) *A Life Together: The Distribution of Attitudes Around the Disabled.* London: Tavistock.

Diehl L W (1976) Changes in popular attitudes to epilepsy in the Federal Republic of Germany and the USA. In: *Epileptology, Proceedings of the 7th International Symposium on Epilepsy,* Janz D (ed.), pp. 97–100. Stuttgart: George Thieme Verlag.

Garrison W M and Tesch S (1978) Self concept and deafness: a review of research literature. *Volta Review,* **80**: 457–466.

Locker D (1983) *Disability and Disadvantage: The Consequences of Chronic Illness.* London: Tavistock.

Scambler G and Hopkins A (1986) Being epileptic: coming to terms with stigma. *Sociology of Health & Illness,* **8**(1): 26–43.

Van Wessem G C (1976) Certain aspects of lay organisations – the situation in Italy. In: *Epileptology, Proceedings of the 7th International Symposium on Epilepsy,* Janz D (ed.), pp. 112–116. Stuttgart: George Thieme Verlag.

Chapter 5

LIVING WITH A
NEUROLOGICAL DISEASE

Chapter theme

A patient who has been told his diagnosis needs some factual information to enable him to protect his personal identity. If he asks the nurse when, where and how often a disease occurs, she can, by consulting the 'Epidemiology' section, place his disorder in a global context; that will help him to realise that he has not just been 'picked out' but is one of many other people similarly affected.

The pressure of work can sometimes make one so hurried that explanations to patients are not so much brief as nonexistent. People need to know why they are asked to undergo special tests and the nurse's ability to provide a factual explanation of the reasons for the tests will help to alleviate fear of the unknown. The detailed description of what happens during the tests is given by doctors or technicians who carry them out, but the nurse should know, and be able to explain in general terms, what is involved (see 'Investigations').

The only way by which a nurse can discover how patients experience the onset and gradual progression of a neurological disorder, leading up to the climax of the diagnosis, is in her conversations with them, sometimes retrospectively. Selected snapshot views of 'Patients' experiences' illustrate the asymptomatic patient, a remitting or persistent condition or the person whose symptoms are alleviated.

Contents

Epidemiology

Patients and relatives will ask 'How often does the disease occur, who gets it and where does it occur?' Some people will be helped by knowing that many others also suffer from their condition, some will feel special by learning that their condition is relatively uncommon. However, everyone enquiring about the epidemiology of a disorder will be relieved to find that the nurses involved in their care possess the knowledge to answer the questions. Epidemiological studies are concerned with the frequency of disease and its predilections by race, sex, age, geography and other features, as well as with the severity and course of the illness. The subject was originally restricted to epidemics of infectious diseases but is now applied generally in medicine and public health.

There are two common methods of expressing the frequency with which a disease occurs in a given population: the *incidence*, the number of new cases recorded every year, and the *prevalence*, the number of cases of a disease present at a given time. The *point prevalence rate* is a ratio and refers to the number of those affected at one point of time within the community. *Mortality* or death rate refers to the number of deaths attributable to a disease within a specified time period and population and is usually given as an annual death rate per 100 000 population. Incidence, mortality and prevalence are all ordinarily expressed in unit-per-population values: for example, 10 cases among a community of 20 000 represents a rate of 50 per 100 000 population, or 0.5 per 1000 population. Table 5.1 shows incidence and point prevalence rates for a variety of neurological conditions (data from Kurtzke, 1984).

Migraine

About 10 per cent or more of the population suffer from migraine at some time and there is often a family history of similar disorder. The female to male ratio is three to two (Cull, 1985).

Epilepsy

Epilepsy is the most common neurological disorder affecting people of all ages. The incidence of epilepsy (non-febrile seizures) in a general population has been estimated at 20–50 cases per 100 000 per year. Most studies have found a slightly higher incidence among males. Fits tend to start in infancy or by late adolescence but the incidence rises again after the age of 65 (Shorvon, 1984; Jeavons and Aspinall, 1985).

Dementia

The fourth most common cause of death in Western society, organic dementia of the Alzheimer type represents one of the major health problems of our time. It has been estimated that 5–10 per cent of the population aged over 65 years suffer from some degree of dementia and the proportion rises to 20 per cent over the age of 80. About 60

Table 5.1 *Neurological conditions – incidence and point prevalence rates*

Annual incidence per 100 000 population

Herpes zoster	400
Migraine	250
Other severe headache	200
Brain trauma	200
Acute cerebrovascular disease	150
Other head injury	150
Epilepsy	50
Dementia	50
Menière's disease	50
Polyneuropathy	40
Transient ischaemic attacks	30
Parkinsonism	20
Subarachnoid haemorrhage	15
Blindness	15
Benign brain tumour	10
Deafness	10
Malignant primary brain tumour	5
Metastatic cord tumour	5
Trigeminal neuralgia	4
Multiple sclerosis	3
Motor neurone disease	2
Guillain Barré syndrome	2
Benign primary cord tumour	1
Huntington's chorea	0.4
Wilson's disease	0.1
Malignant primary cord tumour	0.1

Point prevalence rates per 100 000

Migraine	2000
Other severe headache	1500
Epilepsy	650
Acute cerebrovascular disease	600
Menière's disease	300
Dementia	250
Parkinsonism	200
Transient ischaemic attacks	150
Herpes zoster	80
Multiple sclerosis	60
Benign brain tumour	60
Trigeminal neuralgia	40
Metastic brain tumour	15
Benign primary cord tumour	15
Motor neurone disease	6
Malignant primary brain tumour	5
Metastic cord tumour	5
Huntington's chorea	5
Myasthenia gravis	4
Guillain Barré syndrome	1
Wilson's disease	1

per cent of demented patients have Alzheimer's disease and the proportion increases with age (Harding, 1985).

Parkinson's disease

The 60–80 000 people afflicted with Parkinson's disease in England and Wales make up perhaps 1 per cent of the population over 50 years old. Males and females are equally affected, but light-skinned races are affected more than Negroes (Parkes, 1985).

Multiple sclerosis (MS)

Multiple sclerosis (sometimes known as disseminated sclerosis or DS) usually starts between the ages of 10 and 50 and is slightly more common in females than males. In 8 per cent of patients with multiple sclerosis another family member is affected. Forsythe (1988) explains, 'There seems to be some sort of genetic protection against the disease as shown by the low incidence in certain ethnic groups such as the Japanese, Maoris, Eskimos, the black population of Africa, Australian Aborigines and Indians.'

The most striking epidemiological finding is that the prevalence of the disease is high in northern Europe (latitude 43°N–65°N) and in North America (37°N–52°N), decreasing towards the equator. Individuals who migrate from high to low risk areas acquire a lower prevalence if they migrate before the age of 15 but retain the high risk if they migrate after that age, suggesting that an environmental factor operates in childhood. Epidemics of the disease seem to have occurred in Iceland and the Faroe Islands. The nature of the environmental agent implicated by these epidemiological studies is unknown. Occasionally, viruses have been seen and cultured from MS tissue but, despite the use of very sensitive methods, no single conventional virus can regularly be recovered (Compston, 1985).

Brain tumour

Cerebral glioma is the tenth most frequent malignant tumour in males, while other brain tumours are exceedingly rare. The absolute incidence may be estimated at between 5–15 per 100 000 per year but many small benign tumours may remain undiagnosed in life (Thomas, 1985). (See also Chapter 3.)

Huntington's chorea

Huntington's chorea is one of the most serious genetic disorders of adult life: patients are usually ill for 15 to 20 years. The age of onset is generally about 35 to 40 years, although symptoms can appear earlier or later. There are about 4000 patients with this autosomal dominant condition in Great Britain. It may be more common in parts of the United States, where it was taken by East Anglian migrants who landed in Salem, Massachusetts, in 1632. Some patients are said to have the blue eyes and prematurely grey hair of the original stock (Parkes, 1985). There is no evidence that Huntington's chorea has declined in recent years, despite enhanced awareness of the disorder and the greater availability of genetic counselling.

Motor neurone disease

Prevalence is about 5 per 100 000, the disease usually beginning between the ages of 50 and 70, although it can occur at any age. Males are affected more than females. The disease is distributed uniformly around the world. In the United States more white than non-white patients are affected (Kurtzke, 1982).

Movement disorders

Although Gilles de la Tourette syndrome is a rare disorder, misdiagnosis, the need to survey large populations to obtain accurate statistics and the reluctance of many patients and their families to cooperate fully with research have hampered data collection. Several new cases, most of whom have never been correctly diagnosed, are usually identified after a mass media discussion of Gilles de la Tourette. The syndrome occurs in all races and is distributed equally among different social classes. All the larger series report a male:female incidence of at least three to one, nearly all cases beginning before the age of 12. Spasmodic torticollis occurs equally commonly in the two sexes and has a peak incidence in the fourth decade of life. The peak age of onset of Meige's syndrome is in the sixth decade of life. More women than men are affected by both blepharospasm and Meige's syndrome. The commonest age of presentation of writer's cramp is between 20 and 50 years, with a peak incidence in the third and fourth decades of life. It seems likely that the advent of dictaphones and typewriters has reduced the overall frequency of this disorder to a considerable degree (Lees, 1985).

Investigations

Before the test

Some but not all patients will wish to be informed about the investigations they are to have and they will gain considerable benefit from a suitable explanation. Just how much information or psychological support is needed by the patient undergoing an investigation depends on the individual's previous experiences, personality and anxiety level. A combination of tact, careful attention to verbal and non-verbal communication, and the nurse's own experience of talking to patients will help her to evaluate the patient's information needs. Patients who find that those who are caring for them recognise their fears will be less frightened than those surrounded by insensitive, uncommunicative nurses. The leaflets that many hospitals give to people making test appointments usually satisfy their information needs: the nurse's role is to be alert to any anxieties that patients may have about a forthcoming test, to offer factual information when appropriate and, most importantly, to inform the relevant department of any specific fears expressed by patients.

Patients' questions

The nurse should be prepared to answer a variety of questions requiring factual information, which can be found in this book, in other texts cited, in the patient's medical history and from professional colleagues. Examples of questions include:

Exactly what is the test?
Is the test absolutely necessary?
What degree of pain or discomfort is involved?
Must I prepare for the test in any way?
How does it help to determine the diagnosis?
How will the information obtained influence my treatment?

Patients' fears

Merely acknowledging the unpleasantness of an experience demonstrates the nurse's awareness of fears surrounding unfamiliar events and places.

Why should I have to see frightening equipment?
Will they tell me what's happening during the test?
Will X-rays affect my ability to have babies?
I am scared of needles; will I need an injection?
Will it hurt?
Does it produce side-effects?

Neurological investigations

Neurological investigations include:
- Skull X-ray
- Spinal X-ray
- Electroencephalography (EEG)
- Computed tomography (CT)
- Magnetic resonance imaging (MRI)
- Lumbar puncture
- Electromyography (EMG)
- Angiography
- Myelography

Skull X-ray

This X-ray will show whether or not there is evidence of fractures, raised intracranial pressure, pituitary enlargement, bone disease, alteration of skull shape or abnormal calcification.

Spinal X-ray

The spinal X-ray is used to identify vertebral fractures, dislocation or compression and to note areas of bone erosion or unexpected calcification. It will also help to identify abnormal vertebral column curvatures (scoliosis, lordosis, kyphosis) and to demonstrate narrowing of the vertebral canal.

Electroencephalography (EEG)

Electricity can be detected in many parts of the body. An EEG machine amplifies the constantly changing electrical potentials from the brain surface some 100 000 times and by recording these mechanically on a moving paper roll, provides a permanent visual record that can then be interpreted by electrophysiological specialists (Figure 5.1). The EEG is used to supplement information obtained in the clinical examination of patients suffering from:

- episodes of altered consciousness or behaviour – epilepsy, hypoglycaemia;
- infective conditions – encephalitis, cerebral abscess;
- cerebrovascular lesions – transient ischaemic attacks, mass lesions and metabolic disorders.

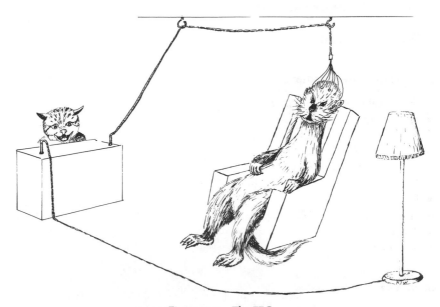

Figure 5.1   The EEG

A variety of recording techniques – for example a routine 1-hour recording, prolonged monitoring with video, or a day or overnight sleep study – may be utilised depending on the clinical problem.

Patients' fears

The fear of electrical shock and pain, or the technician's capacity to read the mind as a result of the test, have all been mentioned by anxious patients. Some people believe that the procedure can indicate whether or not they have mental or emotional illness. Another fear to be on the alert for when discussing investigations with a frightened patient is that the prefix 'electro' reminds a few people of electroconvulsive therapy.

Computed tomography (CT)

This is a non-invasive, safe, painless procedure, conducted with or without the use of a radio-opaque contrast medium, that uses the X-ray beam of a scanner and a computer to provide images of very thin cross-sections of the brain and skull. It shows abnormalities in the size, shape and position of cranial and intracranial structures and differentiates between tumours, haemorrhage and infarction. The advantages of the CT scan are that it is much more sensitive than ordinary X-rays, and high-density structures like bone no longer mask the underlying structures.

Patients' fears

'When the radiologists left me alone in the room, I was frightened, even though they said they were watching through the glass. I wanted to call out to them to come back and let me out.' 'When the scan was finished, I was frightened that they'd leave me there, forget me.'

Magnetic Resonance Imaging (MRI)

If the technique of the 1970s was CT scanning, the technique of the 1980s and beyond is magnetic resonance imaging (MRI, Figure 5.2). It studies how the essential elements of living tissues work, by creating movement in cells through the activity produced by magnetism and radiofrequency energy. Very large magnets, powerful radiofrequency generators and very complex computing systems are required. MRI has the great advantage over X-rays that it uses no harmful ionising radiation and can therefore be used repeatedly without any harmful effect being known to occur. The usefulness of MRI scanning lies in the contrasting of tissues.

Patients' fears

Some patients who suffer from claustrophobia have described the frightening sensation of 'entering a black tunnel' or 'going into a coffin'. The technician who will be looking

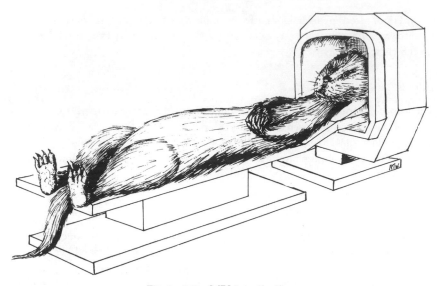

Figure 5.2   MRI investigation

after the patient during the scan must be informed about the patient's expressed or suspected fears, by the nurse or relative who accompanies him.

Lumbar puncture

This procedure is used for obtaining a sample of cerebrospinal fluid (CSF) by puncturing the lumbar meninges below the level of the cord with a long hollow needle inserted between the spines of two lumbar vertebrae.

Normal CSF is clear and colourless like water. Red, yellow or cloudy CSF indicates the presence of blood or leucocytes; abnormal CSF pressure indicates the presence of a space-occupying lesion, infection or dehydration. The number and ratio of cells present can give a guide to possible pathology. The normal protein level of 0.1–0.4 g/l is elevated in most situations in which the meninges are inflamed, where blood has leaked into the cerebrospinal fluid and in multiple sclerosis. There are no blood cells present in healthy CSF, but red cells are found following a subarachnoid haemorrhage and white cells in the patient who has meningitis. Cytological examination of cells will show whether or not they are malignant.

Lumbar puncture procedure is also used to introduce an anaesthetic or dye into the canal for X-ray or myelographical visualisation of the spinal subarachnoid space or other parts of the nervous system.

Headache

The patient should lie flat for 8 to 24 hours afterwards in order to reduce the chance of post-lumbar-puncture headache developing. If a headache does occur bedrest is encouraged for the duration of the pain, with regular simple analgesia if required.

Electromyography (EMG)

Electromyography (EMG) detects, records and interprets the electrical activity occurring in muscle during voluntary contraction or in denervated muscle at rest. The activity can be recorded with needle electrodes inserted into the muscle, amplified and displayed as an auditory signal through a loudspeaker and as a visual signal on an oscilloscope: the signals may be recorded on a magnetic tape or printed out on a paper recorder. Analyses of such electrical activity are important when a diagnosis of muscle disease (myopathies and dystrophies) or lower motor neurone lesions (denervation) is being considered. Tests that measure the speed of conduction in peripheral nerves contribute to the diagnosis of peripheral nerve disorders, particularly those due to local compressive lesions, for example carpal tunnel syndrome.

Angiography

Angiography is the radiographic demonstration of the circulatory system by means of the injection of contrast medium into an artery. In a normal X-ray, the bones are clearly shown and a fracture, for instance, may be demonstrated, but the brain and its blood vessels cannot be seen. If, however, a liquid radio-opaque substance (contrast medium) is injected into the main arteries leading to the brain, it will circulate round the smaller arteries inside the skull, then pass into the capillaries and finally into the veins, so that a composite picture of the cerebral circulation can be built up.

Carotid angiography is used to demonstrate abnormalities of blood supply to the anterior and middle parts of the brain. The abnormalities that can be detected include vessel occlusion, aneurysms, angiomas and clots.

Myelography

Myelography is the radiographic examination of the spinal cord following the injection of radio-opaque contrast medium into the subarachnoid space, usually by way of a lumbar puncture. Myelography identifies the position of the intervertebral discs, spinal cord, nerve roots and identifies any blockage of the canal by tumour or other spinal conditions. A water-soluble dye is widely used, which is absorbed and excreted. Radiographers may ask the patient not to lie down for the first few hours after the procedure in order to reduce cerebral cortex irritation: by allowing fluid to collect in the sacral area, reducing the amount of fluid moving into intracranial spaces and enabling the medium to be diluted and thus reabsorbed more slowly.

After the test

All patients worry about the results of their tests. They must be told what these are, whether negative or positive, because fear of the unknown is a heavier burden to bear than full knowledge of their illness, however serious that may be. As nurses are closest to patients it is their duty to recognise worries and ensure that whoever requested the test is aware of any specific anxieties that the patient has expressed.

Patients' experiences

Cerebrovascular disease: symptoms alleviated

Russell

In 1960 Russell Ritchie wrote a book in which he eloquently describes his struggles while confined to a wheelchair after having had a cerebrovascular accident. Whenever his wife or his daughter took him out for a walk in the wheelchair it was something of a performance. In the corridor outside his flat there was a small lift into which the wheelchair could fit sideways and just leave room for someone to press the button. But the wheelchair was sometimes quite awkward, and many times an irate passenger on the ground floor kept ringing the lift bell while they tried to force the wheelchair in. Then there were the four or five steps leading out of the building. He says that after such an outing 'By the time my wife or my daughter had done that they were trembling and fit to collapse.' With a lot of physiotherapy and vigorous family support Russell did regain his mobility.

Quentin

Quentin woke from his regular evening sleep in the armchair and found that he had no power in his left hand. Although his wife said that his hand had 'gone to sleep', he was not convinced because there was no pins and needles sensation (paraesthesia). A month later there was an incident at work when he dropped something because of a loss of power in his left hand. The next month the same thing happened again; this time he was also dizzy but recovered after about 7 minutes. On another occasion he lost the power in both his left arm and leg while sitting at the lunch table. Three days later his left leg became weak while he walked in the street with his wife, who prevented him from falling.

By now Quentin decided it was time to visit the doctor to see why he was having these attacks. The neurologist told him that he had had five slight strokes, which, if neglected, could lead to paralysis on his left side. After a week in hospital having investigations, Quentin commenced anticoagulant therapy and was encouraged to continue work, although on a part-time basis, and he was strongly advised to stop smoking.

For the next 2 years Quentin had monthly hospital appointments to monitor his anticoagulant therapy. In the first year he reported various symptoms. First was pain in his right calf, which later spread to his foot, and shortly afterwards he noticed blood in his saliva in the mornings. A few months after this the end of his right big toe was thought to be ischaemic because of pain there, which was relieved by sitting with his foot elevated. Blood tests revealed a continuously high level of fat in his blood and a dietitian advised him to follow a low fat diet with restricted carbohydrate. In the last year of anticoagulant therapy he had no further problems and the biggest disappointment that the onset of transient ischaemic attacks (TIAs) had caused him, was to give up work. Nevertheless, he continued to enjoy a lively social life with his wife as they were both active in local charity work.

Pat

Pat, a 55-year-old woman, had transient loss of vision consisting of a thick grey mist in her right eye six or seven times over a 3-month period, the episodes coming on over a few seconds, lasting for a few more seconds and then passing. She could not say where she was when the attacks started: 'I've not taken time to notice, they just come.' There was no warning, no pain and no attack on the other side. She had had transient ischaemic attacks in a variety of situations so the loss of vision was not related to any particular activity. She had always been active, doing canteen work that meant she had to get up at 5 a.m.

The doctor explained to Pat that she had narrowing of the artery in the neck and not enough blood was getting to her eyes, and though the use of anticoagulants would remove her attacks, it could not prevent a stroke. She needed surgery to remove the cholesterol emboli from the internal carotid artery but her blood pressure would have to be stable before she could undergo this. After an arteriogram Pat was considered fit for surgery; she agreed to have the endarterectomy and had an uneventful post-operative recovery. Within a few months of her operation she had resumed her normal busy life-style, although her latest job did not, fortunately, entail getting up at dawn.

Oliver

Oliver had had repeated attacks of blurred vision in both eyes for 3 years: these lasted a few minutes and occurred two or three times a week and were worse in the right eye. He said he could feel 'everything turning over' and that he was swaying. When driving he suddenly found that he was on the wrong side of the road, but fortunately avoided an accident. This 45-year-old man was admitted to hospital for investigation, and an arteriogram showed mild arteriosclerotic changes in the retinal vessels. Oliver's problems were therefore caused by vertebrobasilar ischaemia causing transient ischaemic attacks and he was started on an anticoagulant therapy regime before he left hospital. For the first 3 years on anticoagulant therapy Oliver had only about three giddy spells, then for the next 4 years intermittent attacks of blurred vision in both eyes, sporadic walking difficulties due to poor balance and occasional nosebleeds (epistaxis). During the next 2 years he attended hospital regularly but had no further problems, his anticoagulant therapy was discontinued and he was able to carry on leading a normal healthy life.

Therapeutic approach – transient ischaemic attacks

How to deal with TIAs is really a matter of preventing subsequent stroke and other vascular diseases. There are various ways of reducing the risk of subsequent stroke development; these include stopping smoking, losing weight if the patient is obese, control of hypertension, antiplatelet therapy, anticoagulant therapy and surgery – endarterectomy (removing the lining of an artery).

Degenerative diseases: asymptomatic

Monica

A young woman visited her doctor because she wished to take out life insurance and a medical report was needed. She explained that 7 years earlier her right leg had become numb and when walking in the street her legs were weak: the condition lasted for a few weeks. The problems in her legs ceased but a few months later her eyesight started to go cloudy and she lost the sight in her right eye for 3 weeks. It recovered completely and she had normal vision in both eyes at the time of her neurological examination. On questioning it emerged that she could not tell the temperature of water when she washed her hands and face in the mornings. She said, 'I think I'm perfectly fit.' Although her experiences of remitting symptoms indicated a 7-year history of multiple sclerosis, the lengthy asymptomatic periods implied a good prognosis.

Degenerative diseases: remission of symptoms

Forsythe

Dr Forsythe describes in her book *Living with Multiple Sclerosis* (1979) how her left leg mysteriously became weak just as she finished her final examinations: this was thought to be due to pressure on a nerve. This weakness cleared up after many weeks of rest but she then had periods of extreme fatigue, which were thought to be due to 'lack of guts'. A few years later, after the birth of her second child, she had a spell of double vision, which an oculist said was due to fatigue and recommended rest. She had another period of weakness of both legs and in her right arm following a minor operation. She was working full time, as well as looking after the children and the house, but she became so exhausted and low that she had to ask for sick leave. She was not examined physically but was admitted to a psychiatric nursing home for a rest and spent the first week asleep, which was regarded as a depressive symptom. A year later, while on holiday, she had great difficulty walking on uneven ground and down cliff paths and was embarrassed by falling over frequently for no apparent reason. Ten years after her first symptom she was told that she had multiple sclerosis and after a short period of denial she exchanged a hectic hospital working environment for a rural general practice. Her invaluable contribution to the multiple sclerosis literature incorporates the sufferer's expertise.

Degenerative diseases: persistent symptoms

Nora

A year before she visited her doctor, a young woman found that her right leg was dragging, causing her to catch her toes on steps. This lasted for 2 weeks. About a month after this she had blind spots in her left eye and, later, in her right eye but there was no pain and it did not interfere with her eyesight or reading. She visited her GP, who suggested that if any new symptoms occurred she should go and see him again. Later that year she had bouts of numbness in her hands, which gradually became worse, and paraesthesia (pins and needles) in her right leg. She was told that these were probably symptoms of multiple sclerosis. When Nora complained of extreme fatigue she was admitted to hospital for assessment and special investigations – lumbar puncture and visually evoked responses – which confirmed the diagnosis. Her main problem at this time was tiredness as she worked full-time, studied for professional examinations and organised the household work.

Nora enjoyed a few months with no new episodes but her legs became so weak that she had to use a frame or sticks to get about, and this was shortly followed by urinary incontinence. The speedy march of her symptoms indicated that Nora had a severe form of multiple sclerosis. Two years after her first symptoms began she had very little power in her legs and used a wheelchair all the time. Her arms were shaky with continuous involuntary movements. Her husband had to feed her, as she was by then unable to use a fork or spoon, and she tipped her cup over if it was too full. Her fingers felt a little numb and her writing had deteriorated. She used intermittent self-catheterisation. She lived in an adapted ground floor flat, and was visited by the district nurse, a home help, her friends and family. Nora has discussed alternatives to living at home and has agreed to ask her general practitioner to arrange for residential nursing home care if she ever feels that this would be preferable to continuing to live at home.

Therapeutic approach – multiple sclerosis

Therapeutic support for the patient with multiple sclerosis concentrates on the patient's general health and nutrition, with medical treatment during acute attacks, for example with steroids, and maintenance of mobility. Prophylactic measures to prevent complications and early treatment of complications if they occur focuses on urinary tract infections, degenerative changes in the spinal column, joints and muscles owing to immobility and spasticity. If psychological problems become apparent, these are treated, and employment should be encouraged for as long as possible.

Osbert

Osbert always enjoyed good health until his forty-second year when he began to have psychological difficulties at home and at work. A year later he developed acute diarrhoea and a slurring of speech. Within a few more months his psychiatric state deteriorated, he cried for no obvious reason and his gait was disturbed as he staggered when walking. He had been a very good tennis player and when his wife, an indifferent player, began to beat him he realised that something was wrong. Shortly after this he was walking slowly and had difficulty with washing and dressing. Two years after his initial symptoms Osbert's intellect had deteriorated and he had very little insight into his condition, with limited conversational ability. All these problems and the knowledge that there were two close relatives who had died in psychiatric hospitals confirmed the diagnosis of Huntington's chorea. Following his initial speech difficulties he had continuous involuntary movements, most evident on rest. His movements were described as chorea – continuous, fleeting, semi-purposeful and involving muscles all over the body.

The medical outlook for Osbert's future was bleak as the progressive degeneration of his nervous system would gradually erode both physical and mental faculties with a life-expectancy of about 12 years. Osbert's family was relieved to find a team of district nurses, a home help and access to a day centre would support them for as long as he could live at home. There was also the possibility of hospice or nursing home care in the future.

Movement disorders: symptoms described

Greta

This 50-year-old woman had had pain behind her left ear for 5 years, and her eyelids tended to droop so that they were closed nearly all day. Her main problem developed later, when she found that her head pulled round to one side very uncomfortably. The only time she could keep her head still was when she sat with a cushion behind her head. After 4 years of this embarrassing condition Greta's head adopted an almost fixed position to the side. Although she was otherwise mobile, this focal dystonia caused her problems when crossing the road as she could only easily watch for traffic in one direction but then had to turn her body round to be able to see the other. She was unable to read, write or even watch television because she could not hold her neck up. When she was examined it was observed that her left shoulder was higher than the right because of the constant pulling on the neck muscles. As neither the pathology nor physiology of torticollis is known, a range of drugs acting on central neurotransmitter function may be tried; in Greta's case an anticholinergic drug brought considerable relief.

Hanna

Hanna, a 30-year-old woman, described how she had for many years made uncontrollable noises that were triggered by fast action on television, such as a gunfight, and were worst of all when she was about 15 years old: she found herself repeating phrases from television seconds later (echolalia). She made up words and just shouted them out, not as part of any conversation. This was accompanied by flinging her arms around. When she walked she sometimes dragged one foot. She also often used to grind her teeth, so much so that she found people were staring at her. When worried or tired, for example before examinations, her Gilles de la Tourette syndrome symptoms worsened, but were least likely to occur when she was interested in and concentrating on something. Within 2 weeks after starting to take sulpiride (Dolmatil) she only had some eye-blinking and shoulder-shrugging and her condition would be well controlled in the future with careful monitoring of whichever neuroleptic drug was best for her.

Isaac

Isaac said that as a child he was a constant source of embarrassment to his family because he swore continuously as an effect of the Tourette syndrome. Without any warning he would suddenly produce an uncontrollable string of obscenities. At school teachers had criticised and ridiculed him, and when told to keep quiet he would echo the words spoken to him (echolalia). Occasionally upon command he would stop jumping around. His classmates occasionally ostracised and made a scapegoat of him and he felt rejected: they called him 'the nutty one'. Occasionally, he would let out a sound like a puppy or dog barking, then he would make skipping movements while his head would bob up and down. Public travel was agonising, as the symptoms made him the centre of attention. He could no longer go to the library since vocalisations were not tolerated there. After 10 days in hospital a medication regime of neuroleptic drugs was worked out. He was soon able to travel and visit public places without suffering from socially embarrassing symptoms.

Therapeutic approach – Gilles de la Tourette syndrome

A dramatic improvement for the outcome of the Gilles de la Tourette syndrome occurred with the discovery 20 years ago that haloperidol led to a significant and often dramatic alteration of the symptomatology experienced by patients. It is generally acknowledged to bring relief of tics in 80 or 90 per cent of patients. Some patients with a severe disorder do remarkably well on a small amount of one of the neuroleptic drugs, while others require very large doses. Treatment does not have to go on continually. For many patients the judicious administration of the right drug at a time of increasing disability can then be stopped and the patient can remain treatment-free until the next exacerbation occurs.

Involuntary movements: symptoms alleviated

Harry

Harry, 45 years old, explained that during his adolescence he had made grunting noises and explosive utterances and repeated noises he had heard. He also had a compulsion to touch things and count before he walked. At 38 he noticed that he had involuntary movements of his face. He said that his movements created an inner tension – 'It will explode out' – and his muscles felt torn and tense. When concentrating intensely or while he was sleeping the tics would disappear but they always came back again. His medication kept the movements and noises under control for most of the time so that he was able to work and lead a normal life provided that he remembered to take his neuroleptic drug pimozide (Orap) and kept in contact with the specialist who was treating him for the Gilles de la Tourette syndrome.

Joan

Sixteen years previously 51-year-old Joan had had head turning and blinking, which later developed into a series of constant movements in other parts of her body; there were no obvious trigger factors. Four years after this she developed repeated biting movements. Her head-turning tended to pull to the right. She was diagnosed as suffering from Meige's syndrome, with dystonia of the facial muscles and choreiform movements in limbs. Because of the constant biting movements, she developed dental problems, with root abscesses on all the lower teeth, which had to be extracted. She spent a month in hospital; treatment with an anticholinergic drug, benztropine (Cogentin), proved to be very effective and she was discharged with an improved quality of life ahead of her.

Frank

A 58-year-old left-handed architect with Parkinson's disease found his handwriting was becoming illegible, especially when fine lettering was required, but his drawing skill was unaffected. He had a problem turning taps and could not get the car into first gear; sometimes he had to ask his wife to do up his buttons. Frank had not noticed any trembling in his hands but his general practitioner did observe that his left hand was tremulous. He had lost weight and said, 'I seem to have shrunk', even though he was eating well. He was advised not to give up his professional work or his leisure activities. It was not until 2 years after his initial consultation that he required an anticholinergic drug, benzhexol (Artane). When he retired a few years prematurely he was able to enjoy his leisure interests as the symptoms were well controlled by medication.

Frederick

A 63-year-old man had a slowly progressive tremor in the right hand, especially when writing, shaving and doing up buttons, but it was absent when he was asleep or relaxed. About a year later the tremor in his right leg started. As he explained, 'I feel I'm trembling inside, like the limb is vibrating.' Of walking, he said, 'I've got to keep my mind on walking, unsure if I'm going to make a step or not . . . I'm not as steady as I was, walking or turning round'. He felt that the worst part of his condition was the inconvenience and embarrassment it caused. The symptoms of Parkinson's disease can occur in different degrees: with him the tremor was most marked. By taking carefully regulated dopaminergic drugs, Madopar and Sinemet, and using various aids for dressing and coping at home, he was able to do most of the things he wanted, except when he became self-conscious about his tremor. However, he learnt some practical solutions such as carrying a shopping bag or a rolled-up newspaper or sitting on the offending hand in order not to distract the people he was trying to impress.

Lesley

Lesley, a self-employed businessman who travelled long distances, consulted a doctor because he had difficulty in walking as his left leg was trailing. He was given a dopaminergic drug, which worked immediately, and he was able to continue a normal life style. Later on, his health gradually deteriorated as continuous choreic movements developed; he was a bit stiff first thing in the morning and unable to walk properly. It seemed that he needed tablets more often than the 4-hourly period prescribed. Originally his 8 a.m. tablet made 'the strength flow through him', but gradually it began to take effect later in the day. By 11 a.m. the choreic movements had started and were then relieved by the next dose at 12 noon. By 4 p.m. he was shaking and this continued throughout the evening. He was stiff only in the morning. When asked which was the worst, early morning stiffness or the continuous movements, he said that the movements were embarrassing because people would stare at him.

His movements were choreic because he was in a state of continuous drug intoxication. If the dopaminergic drug were to have been discontinued the choreic movements would have completely disappeared, but there was a risk that Lesley could have become completely immobilised by the Parkinson's disease. A few years later, Lesley was keen to try additional treatment and a different dopaminergic drug was added to his medication; the physiotherapist helped him to develop some useful exercises and techniques to improve his posture and gait.

Therapeutic approach – Parkinson's disease

Parkinson's disease is caused by degeneration and loss of the neurones in the substantia nigra. These neurones are dopaminergic – they produce and release the neurotransmitter dopamine. The control of voluntary movement is dependent on a balance between the two neurotransmitters dopamine (DA) and acetylcholine (ACh). In Parkinson's disease there is a deficiency of dopamine because of the destruction of the dopaminergic neurones and the balance between ACh and DA is disturbed; the symptoms of the disease result. Treatment of the disease is therefore aimed at producing a normal balance between ACh and DA.

Anticholinergic drugs block cholinergic receptors and therefore decrease the effect of ACh and allow a more normal balance between ACh and DA to be achieved. Some drugs increase dopamine levels and others act directly at the dopamine receptors and mimic the activity of dopamine at the receptor. Other drugs act by increasing the normal synthesis of dopamine and increasing the rate of release of dopamine from the dopaminergic neurone, or by inhibiting the enzyme responsible for the destruction of dopamine. Anticholinergic drugs are most effective against rigidity, tremor and increased salivation, but have little effect on bradykinesia. Occasionally the transformation from involuntary movements and mobility to profound Parkinsonism is so abrupt that patients liken the experience to the operation of an internal switch, and the term 'on–off' syndrome is used.

Katya

One day when out walking in the garden Katya fell but was able to get back to the house and have her tea; she then developed pain in the left side of her face. She went to many doctors in different specialties but none could help her. Three years after the fall she noticed that the left side of her mouth was pulled down and the monthly tension headaches that she had had for 3 years began to occur daily and spread from her head to her face and neck. Seven years later she developed pain in her left upper gum, which gradually got worse: by this time it was clear that she was suffering from unilateral Meige's syndrome. Reading, sewing and watching television were all difficult because the pain was all over her face, mostly in her eyes. Her face felt as 'though it's stuck together': the muscles felt tight. The blepharospasm prevented her from keeping her eyes open and all she could do was to sit down with her eyes closed. She had to leave her job as a cashier because she could no longer see the till. She blinked frequently and had greasy skin, a tender forehead and contraction of the left sternomastoid muscle, which almost continuously pulled her mouth towards the left.

During a short spell in hospital an anticholinergic drug was tried with poor response but, later, a combination of this and dopaminergic antagonists relieved some of her symptoms. A few sessions of acupuncture were tried but these only brought relief for a day or two. Finally, 12 years after her problems first began, she responded well to a course of botulinum toxin injections into the left sternomastoid muscle and, apart from brief attacks of pain in her gum, she was relieved of all the spasms and involuntary facial movements that had tormented her for so long.

Linda

One day, Linda, a 45-year-old woman, felt tension building up in her head, although there was nothing special or significant about the day on which it began. In the next few months her head kept pulling to the left side – it got worse until, eventually, her head remained fixed in one position. Within a year she had to give up working. Ten years after the onset of her torticollis the neck twisting changed – her head pulled backwards as well as to the side. There were no remissions, but the twisting increased when she walked or was in any stressful situation. None of the anticholinergic and benzodiazepine drugs she was given had helped, nor did a course of acupuncture. Linda was one of the first lucky patients to receive effective treatment with botulinum toxin injected into the affected sternomastoid and splenius capitus muscles. Apart from mild dysphagia lasting a few hours after her first injection, there were no ill effects. Linda attended hospital for injections of 1.5 ml of the solution into two separate sites of each selected muscle. Within a week of her first treatment she was able to control her neck position and the pain that she had been experiencing in previous months completely disappeared. Having completed one course of treatment with three hospital treatments, Linda was very happy and accepted that she might need further treatment in the future.

Intracranial tumours: symptoms alleviated

Sheila

The first thing that Sheila noticed was a funny sensation on the bottom left side of her lip. This numbness spread to the left inside of her mouth, her cheek and then her head. She had slight noises in her left ear (tinnitus) and mild unsteadiness – when walking she veered slightly towards the left but she was able to concentrate to stop this. She said that sometimes her hearing was a bit 'muffled' on the left but this did not bother her. When this 53-year-old woman was examined she missed some light cotton-wool touches in all three (ophthalmic, maxillary and mandibular) divisions of the Vth cranial nerve, and a mild hearing loss on the left was identified on audiometry. A CT scan had to be enhanced before an acoustic neuroma became clearly visible. The aim of treatment was to remove the tumour while it was small and before facial asymmetry, complete eye closure and disturbances of other cranial nerves occurred. It was very important for all the implications of surgery to be explained to her. Postoperative difficulties could affect her swallowing, balance and hearing, and could leave her with left-sided facial weakness as well as a tarsorrhaphy, in which the eyelids are stitched together to protect the cornea when the facial VIIth cranial nerve is damaged in surgery. She agreed to have surgery and postoperatively had a mild facial weakness, which improved: she had no further tinnitus, unsteadiness when walking nor numb sensations on her face.

Susan

Susan, 40 years of age, lived alone. Her family noticed that she appeared to be rather depressed and had lost her appetite, and persuaded her to seek medical advice. They told the doctor that 5 years earlier Susan had lost her self-confidence when she was made redundant from a good job; subsequently she got into financial difficulties, something which was new to her. Two years later she had fallen and cut her head sufficiently to require several sutures. Since then she explained that her vision was 'not quite right' and when she began to stumble it was because she 'couldn't see properly, but didn't want to trouble anyone'. When Susan eventually did attend her family doctor she was found to have severe loss of vision and it seemed curious that she had failed to report this herself. When asked, she admitted that in recent months she had noticed some changes in her memory.

She had had no menstrual periods for 2 years (amenorrhoea), her skin was dry and her reflexes were slow. Hypothyroidism was confirmed by blood tests and a very large pituitary tumour was seen on the CT scan. The tumour was removed surgically and although she did not get her vision back in the left eye, her right eye improved; hormonal replacement helped her to regain some of her former good health and spirits.

Rosemary

Rosemary, a 38-year-old woman, woke up every night with nausea and vomiting. The pressure headaches she was getting occurred in different parts of her head. She felt as if she were pregnant with morning sickness, despite having had a hysterectomy. She had a slight speech problem and would lose her train of thought. A few months before coming to hospital she left her car in the wrong place, which was very unusual for her. One day at breakfast she was unable to find the spoon on her left side. She was unsafe when crossing the road. She noticed that she had double vision, her thoughts raced ahead of her and she became forgetful and irritable. Her difficulty increased while she was in hospital: despite being given directions she could not find her way, lost her bed, and she spent an entire morning looking for her hairbrush. Upon examination she was found to have a left hemianopia and marked topographical disorientation (inability to find her way in familiar surroundings). It was also noticed that she had speech problems and dribbled from the left side of her mouth. She had also made errors in simple calculations and with simple general knowledge facts.

A scan showed a right-sided parietal lobe tumour; when it was removed surgically the histological examination identified a malignant lymphoma. Postoperatively she had some facial weakness. A short course of steroids reduced the cerebral oedema, the hemianopia resolved and the headaches were much less severe, although she still had problems in finding her way about. Rosemary was prescribed a 5-week course of radiotherapy postoperatively to diminish residual tumour bulk and decrease the risk of late recurrence.

Intracranial tumours: living for today

Ronald

The first thing 65-year-old Ronald noticed was that 'things wouldn't fit into place'. He explained that he stammered a lot, something he had never done before. He could understand most but not all of what was said to him. When reading he would get so far with a sentence and then could go no further. His wife told the doctor that she had found difficulty understanding him because of his speech problem.

When the doctor examined Ronald he found a dense right-sided hemianopia. A CT scan indicated a lesion deep in the occipitoparietal region, which was thought to be a glioma. He was given a course of steroids to reduce cerebral oedema. A biopsy confirmed that it was a glioma and his steroids were continued in a low dose for several months, over which time he remained stable. Unfortunately malignant cerebral glioma carries a dismal prognosis, depending on grade, in spite of treatment.

Stephen

A retired butcher who had always been physically active was up a ladder working on a tree when the ladder slipped and he fell. About a week later he had a tight feeling at the back of his skull and pins and needles down his left arm, followed by jerking movements, which his wife could not restrain: these attacks lasted from 5 to 20 minutes and occurred about six times. The attacks were focal motor seizures affecting his arm. Since then his arm became stiff and later it became 'frozen'. A chest X-ray showed the presence of carcinoma of the bronchus.

After experiencing continuous pain in the back of his neck for some 10 weeks, Stephen had further investigations and his CT scan indicated that carcinoma secondaries were present in the parietal lobe. The worry was that this was the first of many such lesions. A right frontal craniotomy was performed for total removal and evacuation of a cyst, which was metastatic. He had no postoperative complications and a short course of deep X-ray therapy was given afterwards, but the prognosis was as dismal as it had been for Ronald.

Intracranial tumours: nature wins

Rebecca

Fifty-five-year-old Rebecca was in a supermarket one day in January when she collapsed with what was described by the ambulance man who attended her as an epileptic seizure. Three weeks before the seizure her left hand was getting clumsy, she had lost her appetite and had intermittent headaches. Her husband said that she had some memory problems and slurred speech and he had noticed that her housework had deteriorated; she had found it extremely difficult to organise the family for Christmas. As soon as she was admitted to hospital a CT scan was performed; overnight she became progressively drowsy, her right pupil was larger than the left, indicating compression of the optic nerve, and she was given steroids to reduce cerebral oedema. She was taken to theatre and a biopsy identified that Rebecca had a Grade III astrocytoma; this was treated with radiotherapy and steroids. She improved initially, her headache resolved and there was some improvement in the power of her left hand. She was treated with anticonvulsants. Six months later, her symptoms recurred, she became comatose and died soon after.

Pain: symptoms alleviated

Ann

A young woman complained of severe headaches and dizzy spells in which her head felt as though it was spinning and she felt very sick: she explained that she had slight dizziness all the time. The severe episodes, with thumping pain in her ear and neck, were frightening. Physical examination revealed no neurological abnormalities and Ann was told that she was normal, and that her headaches were caused by muscular tension in the head and neck. The doctor was keen to make Ann realise that he knew she was suffering from headaches and that he was not 'accusing her of being mad'. Ann was advised to use simple analgesics and ice packs regularly to prevent the attacks. The time that was spent by Ann talking about her tension headaches, learning that they were not due to an abnormality of structure nor a threat to her general health and that help was available whenever she should need it, all contributed to the alleviation of her symptoms.

Betty

For 2 years, Betty, a businesswoman, had had continuous throbbing headaches, which were worst across her eyes. The throbbing would suddenly worsen until it was all over her head, and within a couple of hours would become very severe: sometimes it made her sick and she would have to lie down in the staff room. Her mouth felt 'funny' and her lips and tongue felt swollen; her cheek tingled, mostly on the left side, following the headache – this lasted for up to 3 hours and she then found it hard to talk. People noticed several times a week that her speech was slurred. Nothing brought on the attacks; prior to medication the only thing that helped was going to bed. Painkillers particularly designed to treat migraine got rid of the bad headache and tingling.

The doctor explained that her tension headache was physiologically like spraining a wrist – the muscle is tight, the swelling and tenderness causes more muscle tension and a vicious cycle occurs – this was why she had a background headache all the time. She was advised to take 2 weeks off work to rest at home, with a prescription of a compound prophylactic drug, propanolol, and an analgesic to remove the background pain, while the swelling was relieved with an ice pack. The prophylactic medication had to be taken daily, regardless of whether or not she was in pain at the time. It was 6 weeks before the number and severity of her attacks was reduced, but 3 months later she was able to discontinue all medication and remained pain-free for the next year of monitoring.

Bob

This patient, who suffered from cluster headaches, described two different kinds of pain: the pain in his head, which he called migraine, and that on his face, which he called neuralgia. Both types of pain occurred at the same time each day and he had no idea what brought them on. The longer they lasted, the worse they became. The headaches occurred in bouts or clusters lasting for up to 3 months, with headache-free intervals between bouts lasting for a few months. His wife noticed that during a headache period his face was tender and it looked puffy. Because of the severity of the pains he had regularly to get up at 3 or 4 a.m. but they always returned an hour after he went back to bed. He would then get up again and not bother to go back to bed. 'It's a pain out of this world, I could put my head in the oven.' He was successfully treated with an antihistamine that is structurally related to the tricyclic antidepressants – pizotifen (Sanomigran).

Therapeutic approach – headache

The patients who are referred to the specialist are those with intractable, frequent or severe attacks. Radical changes in an active person's life-style are rarely feasible. However, minor adjustments may curtail the body's need to enforce a rest from the hurly-burly by means of a migraine attack. Treatment that is successful for one patient may not be for another with the same symptoms. Equally, successful treatment may fail at some later date in the same patient. Remissions and exacerbations may or may not occur and placebos may be effective for a period and then fail. Thus a flexible approach is needed in the management of these conditions.

Carl

For 7 years, Carl had had attacks of right facial pain, which usually lasted for days or weeks with long intervals of freedom. The pain had now become more severe, persisting for days at a time, and the attacks occurred more frequently. In each attack the pain started in his right cheek and spread to his forehead; sometimes his eye watered. On occasions when the pain was bad the eye closed up but there was neither redness nor discharge. There were times when the pain persisted all day; there were no trigger factors that he could identify. He managed to get to sleep but sometimes the pain woke him at night. He had tried cold and hot compresses, but neither had helped. Carl was suffering from migrainous neuralgia. Initially he was treated with steroids and a few weeks later he was given propranolol, a betablocker, to prevent further attacks. After a year on this regime he was able to discontinue his medication and remained pain-free.

Doreen

Doreen had multiple sclerosis. She attended hospital in order to find out what was causing attacks of stabbing pain that lasted 5 minutes and occurred several times a day. The slightest movement could trigger the pain, so that when she ate the pain started on the left side of her face and shot up to her ear in a sudden jab. She felt as though her face was about to explode, that it was like being struck by lightning. She lost 6 stone in weight in 3 years and she became depressed and suicidal with the pain. This was a severe case of trigeminal neuralgia occurring in brief paroxysms unilaterally, the side of her face later becoming numb as well as continuously in pain. She underwent a medullary tractotomy to divide the nerve fibres in the medulla and midbrain that triggered the pain. She was very pleased to be free of pain and began to gain weight.

Elizabeth

Elizabeth, 70 years old, overweight and hypertensive, suffered from degenerative joint disease (osteoarthritis) affecting the cervical and lumbar spine, knees, hands, wrists and feet. She visited her GP regularly to have her blood pressure checked and her various medications for hypertension and rheumatic pains monitored. When she complained of a dull ache in her right hand and forearm, which was most severe during the night, this might have been thought to be just another rheumatic problem, but the ache was getting worse and she was particularly disturbed by pain in the base of her right thumb. She described the pain as numb, worse in the thumb and adjacent fingers but travelling to the wrist and lower forearm. She was awakened by the pain during the night and would shake her hand to try to relieve the symptoms. When the doctor examined her hands he found that both thumb base joints were stiff, tender and painful during movement and that there was wasting of both thenar eminences: this indicated carpal tunnel syndrome. Elizabeth was cured by a minor operation – a complete section of the ligament.

Myasthenic disorders: symptoms alleviated

Patricia

When Patricia was 16 years old, people noticed that her right eyelid was 'hanging down'. It was worse on some evenings because of muscle fatigue but on many days the problem did not occur at all. She could not breathe deeply at sport and her voice would fade out when reading. Twelve months later, when she had a cold and could neither swallow nor cough, she collapsed and was taken to hospital where she had to be intubated: a diagnosis of myasthenia gravis was made and she commenced anticholinesterase therapy. Three years later she had a thymectomy, which produced a remission in her myasthenia gravis: her youth and the quick response to surgical treatment suggested that she would gradually no longer need the anticholinesterase tablets and that she could anticipate a normal healthy life-style in the future.

Rosemary

Rosemary, a needlework student, had had double vision and fatigue for several months: this did not worry her unduly as it seemed likely that these symptoms were the result of eye strain and long hours of standing at her easel. Soon, however, more alarming symptoms began to appear – when she was ironing a dress she suddenly found that she could not hold up her head, which kept dropping forward uncontrollably. Shortly after this her knees started to give way under her, especially after running and often on dismounting from her bicycle. Her eyelids would droop uncontrollably when she was tired – far more than in ordinary sleepiness – and after sewing for a while her arm would drop to her side. And so it was with all forms of muscular exertion: she would just feel weak, and have to stop and rest. After a short while she would feel her strength returning and be able to carry on – she felt that her muscles were perfectly strong yet she could not make them respond to her will. By this time she was badly frightened but she tried hard to swallow her fear and fight the symptoms because she hated the thought of having to leave college. Rosemary's parents insisted that she should have medical attention. After recovering from the initial shock of learning that their daughter's symptoms were caused by a disease with an alarming name, myasthenia gravis, the future looked brighter as Rosemary responded quickly to steroid medication and a thymectomy, indicating that the disease could be well controlled. After completing her studies Rosemary got a job restoring tapestries in a museum.

Therapeutic approach – myasthenia gravis

Modern treatment of myasthenia gravis is successful in returning most patients to productive lives. Four effective approaches to treatment are available: anticholinesterase agents, immunosuppressive drugs, thymectomy and plasmapheresis. The choice of therapy will be determined by such factors as the age of the patient, the severity and duration of symptoms, the response to previous treatment, the presence of a thymoma and the possible relationship to other diseases. Anticholinesterase agents improve neuromuscular transmission but do not correct the basic receptor defect. Thymectomy and adrenal corticosteroids interfere with the autoimmune reaction. The place of thymectomy in long-term treatment of myasthenia gravis is established. There is an increasing tendency to operate on patients at an early stage of the disease as there is no need to wait until drug control is inadequate. The main advantage of thymectomy is the possibility of obtaining permanent improvement.

References

Compston D A S (1985) Demyelinating disease. In: *Neurology*, Ross Russell R W and Wiles C M (eds.), pp. 145–152. London: Heinemann.

Cull R E (1985) Epilepsy, migraine and headache. In: *Neurology*, Ross Russell R W and Wiles C M (eds.), p. 119. London: Heinemann.

Forsythe E (1979) *Living with Multiple Sclerosis*. London: Faber and Faber.

Harding A E (1985) Degenerative disorders. In: *Neurology*, Ross Russell R W and Wiles C M (eds.), p. 189. London: Heinemann.

Jeavons P M and Aspinall A A (1985) *The Epilepsy Reference Book*. London: Harper and Row.

Kurtzke J F (1982) Motor neurone disease. *British Medical Journal*, **284**(1): 141–142.
Kurtzke J F (1984) Neuroepidemiology. *Annals of Neurology*, **16**: 265–277.
Lees A J (1985) *Tics and Related Disorders*. Edinburgh: Churchill Livingstone.
Parkes J D (1985) Extrapyramidal disease and involuntary movements. In: *Neurology*, Ross Russell R W and Wiles C M (eds.), p. 155. London: Heinemann.
Ritchie D (1960) *Stroke: A Diary of Recovery*. London: Faber and Faber.
Shorvon S D (1984) *Epilepsy*. London: Update Publications.
Thomas D G T (1985) Intracranial tumours. In: *Neurology*, Ross Russell R W and Wiles C M (eds.), p. 96. London: Heinemann.

Further reading

Prevalence and incidence – epidemiology

Dean G, Goodall J and Downie A (1981) The prevalence of multiple sclerosis in the Outer Hebrides compared with North East Scotland and Orkney and Shetland Islands. *Journal of Epidemiology and Community Health*, **35**(2): 110–113.
Holland W W, Karhausen L and Wainwright A H (1978) *Health Care and Epidemiology*. London: Henry Kimpton.
Roberts A (1986) Demographic and social aspects of ageing. *Nursing Times*, Systems of Life, **137**(2): 43–46.
Twining T C and Allen D G (1981) Disability factors among residents of old people's homes. *Journal of Epidemiology and Community Health*, **35**(3): 205–207.
Yarnell J W G, Voyle G J, Richards C J and Stephenson T P (1981) The prevalence and severity of urinary incontinence in women. *Journal of Epidemiology and Community Health*, **35**(1): 71–4.

Investigations

Haughey C W (1981) CT scans. *Nursing* (USA), **11**(12): 72–77.
Hounsfield G N (1973) Computerized transverse axial screening (tomography): Part 1. Description of system. *British Journal of Radiology*, **46**(552): 1016–1022.
Hawkins C (1979) Patients' reactions to their investigations: a study of 504 patients. *British Medical Journal*, **2**: 638–640.
Mastaglia F L, Black J L, Cala L A and Collins D W K (1977) Evoked potentials, saccadic velocities, and computerised tomography in diagnosis of multiple sclerosis. *British Medical Journal*, **1**: 1315–1317.
Matthews D (1984) Nuclear magnetic resonance. *Nursing Times*, **80**(29): 36–38.
Sandercock P, Molyneux A and Warlow C (1985) Value of computed tomography in patients with stroke: Oxfordshire Community Stroke Project. *British Medical Journal*, **290**(1): 193–197.
Scott D (1976) *Understanding EEG: An Introduction to Electroencephalography*. London: Duckworth.

Patients' experiences

Cook S (1979) *Ragged Owlet*. London: Arrow Books.
Corbertt A L (1983) Disabling illness: a personal account. *British Medical Journal*, **286**(1): 1403–1404.
Evans M (1978) *A Ray of Darkness*. London: Calder.
Luria A R (1975) *The Man with a Shattered Brain*. Harmondsworth: Penguin Books.
Sacks O (1984) *A Leg to Stand On*. London: Duckworth.
Spark M (1959) *Memento Mori*. London: Macmillan.

INDEX

N.B. Page numbers in *italics* refer to figures and tables